IN THE
BLINK OF
AN EYE

Books by Alan Doelp

Shocktrauma (1980)
Not Quite a Miracle (1983)
Autumn's Children (1985)

IN THE BLINK OF AN EYE

Inside a Children's Trauma Center

ALAN DOELP

PRENTICE HALL PRESS

NEW YORK · LONDON · TORONTO · SYDNEY · TOKYO

While the cases described in this book are based
on real children and their experiences, either
witnessed or studied by the author, they are in
most instances representative composites, so as
to preserve the privacy and anonymity of the
patients and their families.

Prentice Hall Press
Gulf+Western Building
One Gulf+Western Plaza
New York, New York   10023

Library of Congress Cataloging-in-Publication Data

Doelp, Alan.
  In the blink of an eye: inside a children's trauma center / Alan
Doelp.—1st ed.
    p. cm.
  ISBN 0-13-131871-3 : $17.95
  1. Children's Hospital National Medical Center. 2. Pediatric
trauma centers—Washington (D.C.). 3. Pediatric trauma centers—
United States. I. Title.
RJ28.W313D64 1989
362.1'1'09753—dc19   88-25556
                                                                CIP

Manufactured in the United States of America

10 9 8 7 6 5 4 3 2 1

First Edition

For Phil Heisler, who gave me my big break

Acknowledgments _____

The toughest part of writing a book is figuring out where to stop. No book ever presumes to tell the *entire* story, down to the last obscure detail; it is the author and the author alone who has to choose the cutoff point, decide which details go and which stay, which people appear in the book and which ones only get honorable mention in the introduction.

This book was particularly difficult to conclude, because there is no natural stopping place. Every day the legend of the Children's Trauma Center grows larger, adding new faces, new cases, new lives saved. Already the place is recognized as the flagship of the pediatric trauma movement in America; soon people will also know it as the nation's leading advocate of accident prevention.

This does not happen accidentally. The code room team could not function without the help and support of many other individuals whose jobs may be less romantic but are just as important. A good example is Leon Bowman, who inherited the trauma service's computerized database from Tom McGinley and Tony Mangubat. Statistics are the coin of the realm in the trauma business, and Leon has patiently, meticulously transformed a ragged collection of numbers into a powerful electronic picture of three thousand consecutive trauma cases. It is that database, for example, that shows conclusively that the Children's Trauma Center routinely saves the lives of children who, statistically, should not have survived. When Marty Eichelberger sallies forth to do battle in the name of pediatric trauma centers, he goes armed with Leon's numbers. Nor does Leon do it all alone any longer; in the summers, he gets help from Adam Lowenstein, who in addition to being good with computers, plays a ferocious game of Dig-Dug.

Equally vital to the work of the trauma service is Kelly Farrell, who manages the trauma staff office. Kelly has the unenviable job of keeping track of a group of high-strung and fast-moving professionals and making sure messages get through; phone calls get answered; appointments get kept; bills get paid; equipment ordered, installed, and repaired; and so on and on, in ever-changing detail. She is also the prime organizer of the trauma service's legendary Christmas parties. Through it all, she somehow manages to be both efficient and gracious at the same time.

Ceil Hendrickson ought to be in the book; her job is to go out into the communities served by the Children's Trauma Service and explain the service to interested groups and organizations. Her duties could be described as outreach or as education; what she does, on a community level, is much the same as what Herta Feely does, on a national level, with her National Safe Kids Campaign. Both are working to educate parents on the need for safety; they are also helping to ensure that, when something does happen, parents will know what to do, whom to call, where to take an injured child. Ceil's job is to carry that message to the trauma service's local constituency. It is an important job, and by rights it ought to have a chapter in this book. But you have to stop somewhere, and Ceil, who is married to a writer, will understand that better than most.

The pediatric EMS training program would make another book, between the war stories the medics could tell and the genuinely interesting sessions that feature members of the Children's Hospital faculty of teacher-doctors, both of which convey a wealth of information that would be both valuable and interesting to parents. But alas, with so much else to tell, they get only a single chapter.

Herta Feely gets the credit for coming up with the National Safe Kids Campaign, and that is appropriate because she is the up-front spokesperson. But she gets help from Karen Hilder, Deb Clark, David Mitchell, and Nancy Reeder, who handle the day-to-day routine and the not-so-routine, as well.

Many important stories remain untold. I had promised Ron Tobin, who runs the physical plant, that his name would appear in the book in the same sentence as the word *slumlord.* He outfoxed me, though: He moved the trauma staff out of their broom-closet offices and into spacious new digs. Children's Hospital is suffering from its own success, and the never-ending battle for floor space would be humorous if the players were not dead serious about it. Ron lives in the center of that cyclone; it is a tough job. Someday, I'll write a book about it.

Someday I'll write a book about social workers, too. Mirean Coleman gets written about in a little detail, but the others—Trent Lewis, Leslie Strauss, even Hal Lipton—get short shrift. Maybe next time . . .

When I began my research at Children's Hospital, I spent a great deal of time in the Emergency Communications and Information Center, which gets only passing mention in the book. This, too, is an injustice; the ECIC is probably worth a book in itself. It is the nerve center of the operation, the link to the outside world, where the accidents happen. Without the ECIC, the rest of the system would be nearly useless. Nor is Dave Hunter the only ECIC operator, though his is the only name that appears in the book. I spent many an interesting hour in the company of other operators including John Clark, Fred Thomas, Tom Hodge, Alan Graves, Jim Burke, and Lori Rouser, professionals all.

Neither Don Brown nor Dr. Donald Delaney get mentioned in the book, yet without their help the trauma service would never have got off the ground. Don Brown is the CEO at Children's, and before that he was the second in command. He came to Children's from a hospital in Oklahoma that had recently added a trauma program. He had seen all the battles, all the factional infighting, all the professional jealousy, and had made up his mind that the same thing would not be allowed to happen at Children's. And it didn't. This would have been a different book had there been powerful villains lurking in the shadows of power, plotting the downfall of Eichelberger and his trauma service, but no such thing ever happened. There were people who resisted Marty Eichelberger, but Don Brown supported both Marty and his program from the outset, and together they simply steamrollered any opposition. And, as the numbers so unarguably show, that was the right thing to do.

The hospital's institutional commitment to a trauma program might have created bad blood anyway, but for the consummate diplomatic skills of Dr. Donald Delaney, vice-president for medical affairs. Dr. Delaney is the physician Marcus Welby wishes he could have been. After a long and distinguished career as a pediatrician at Children's, Dr. Delaney—at a time when most people would be planning their retirement—instead accepted an administrative job. Now the famous bedside manner that enchanted two generations of children and parents gets applied to soothing bruised egos, smoothing ruffled feathers, and reminding people that whatever is best for the children is also best for the institution.

There is throughout all of Children's Hospital a sort of warmth, a pervasive sense of calm and gentle affection that helps to soothe the hurt and heal the sick. That sort of atmosphere does not happen by accident; it grows by deed and by example of Don Delaney and the hundreds of others like him who work at Children's Hospital because —first, last, and always—they love kids.

The nurses, as ever, are the unsung heroes of the book. Eve Zimmerman was not David Myers's only nurse, but once again, you have to stop somewhere, so for the purposes of this book Eve represents all the dozens of nurses who invested their time, their affection, and a great deal of very hard work in little David Myers—and who all deserve a share of the payoff. Good nursing, like an institutional love of kids, does not happen by accident; were it not for the daily work of people like Maggie Huey and Astrid Ellis in the ER, Cathy McMahon in the ICU, Jo Talley on 4-Blue, and indeed Elaine Frevert, the vice-president for nursing, Children's Hospital would not be such a special place. But Children's is one of the few hospitals in the country that has not been affected by the nursing shortage, a fact that says more about the place, and the nurses there, than a score of books could. It's simple: At Children's Hospital people love kids.

Marty Eichelberger is one of those people. He appears throughout the book, but readers will doubtless wonder why he's not there more, saving lives with his own two hands, carrying out the duties and responsibilities of the archetypal Hero of Medicine. That's not Marty's style. Coaches don't carry the football, any more than generals fight in the trenches. Marty's intent, from the beginning, was to build a system and an organization that would carry out his ideas and achieve his goals far beyond the capability of any one man. He has done that at Children's Hospital, and he is beginning to spread his medical gospel across the nation. No one will ever be able to count the lives saved, directly and indirectly, by the work of Marty Eichelberger. He gets the credit, but the real glory, and what this book is about, is not in the man but in the system.

◆ ◆ ◆

Writing a book is not of the same magnitude as building a trauma center, but nevertheless a lot of infrastructure goes into it.

I wrote most of this book on my trusty old Compucorp 775 word processor, truly one of the finest typing machines ever built. My friends at Systems Associates—Chuck Cavolo, Mike Lutz, Bob Bogar, and Sherrie LeBaron—have bailed me out of so many cybernetic jams over the years that I can't begin to thank them one by one. Suffice it to say that Systems Associates routinely delivers the kind of service that most computer firms only brag about.

But I owe an equal debt of gratitude to Michael Crandell and Mark Zutkoff, who—when I set off for Texas to write part of this book on my little lap-top computer—provided me with a copy of Crandell Development Corp.'s *SunWord,* a truly magnificent piece of second-generation word-processing software. Officially, I was testing the program for them; the truth is that there were no bugs to speak of, only the inspired work of two talented programmers who, like me, grew up on the Compucorp system.

I doubt I will ever write a book without acknowledging the corrupting influence of Jon Franklin, and through him, the ghost of G. Vern Blasdell. Jon taught me that no matter how tough it is, the view is always worth the climb. He was right, of course. I shall never forgive him.

I owe gratitude especially to my mother, who gave me safe haven for several weeks when the project got so overwhelming that I had to run away somewhere to regain my grip on it. Likewise, I am grateful to Carol Benner, who kept my own household running in my absence and who, throughout the two-year effort, valiantly resisted the temptation to help.

Dominick Abel, my agent, believed in the idea; Gareth Esersky bought it; and PJ Dempsey brought it to life. Susan Llewellyn fixed up my punctuation, grammar, spelling, and occasionally my logic, creating the illusion that I did it myself. They will all insist that they were simply doing their jobs; they have my gratitude nevertheless.

The list goes on and on. Dana Levitz, Kelly Gilbert, Dennis Evans, Maggie Huey, Cyndy Wright, and Heidi Zwick pointed out dumb mistakes or answered dumb questions. Most of all, they, and many others, generously understood that writing is a hermit's game and that friendly phone calls are not a kindness. To all those very special friends I am most especially indebted.

Preface

Accidental injury kills eight thousand children every year in the United States. It is not merely the leading cause of death among children, it is overwhelmingly the greatest threat to young lives. Accidental injury kills more children than all other causes combined.

This came as a shock to me. I set out to write about the Children's Hospital National Medical Center simply because it is a wonderful place full of wonderful people who love kids. I had no notion of the magnitude of the problem. Even after I began my research, and watched case after case roll into the code room, I didn't realize how bad the numbers were. The first time Herta Feely threw out the number eight thousand I simply assumed she had gotten it wrong. She hadn't. Eight thousand kids a year die in accidents. That works out to about one an hour.

I was appalled. Polio never killed anywhere near eight thousand kids a year, but in the polio days there was near panic across the country every summer. Mothers marched in the streets and collected dimes to fight off this killer. Eventually a lot of very smart scientists came up with a cure for polio.

Accidental injury is a different sort of problem. Until the Salk vaccine, there was no way to prevent polio; there are lots of ways to prevent accidents.

The airwaves are full of accident prevention messages these days, because Marty Eichelberger and his trauma staff are convinced that they are treating too many hurt kids. Half, maybe more, of all the accidents could have been prevented. So Children's Hospital, with the generous help of the Johnson & Johnson company and the National Safety Council, has started the National Safe Kids Campaign. If it works, they will save more lives a year with advertisements and brochures than they save with all the medical resources of the hospital itself.

But Marty and his team also understand that not all accidents can be prevented. They understand, in intimate and often blood-spattered detail, the desperate need for specialized pediatric trauma centers. Children are not miniature adults; they require special handling and special care when injured. If they don't get it, they can suffer as much damage from the treatment as from the injury. Children's Hospital National Medical Center is a national pioneer in the care of injured children; the trauma service that Marty Eichelberger has built stands as a model for all others.

This book attempts to deal with all the many facets of the Children's Trauma Service, from how it came into being to what it does for the patient and the patient's family. The cases described here are all real, as are most of the names used. Some families did request anonymity, and in those cases I changed not only names but a few other key facts to help disguise them. A few cases are outright composites, amalgams of cases I witnessed and other case histories that I studied. The composite cases allowed me to illustrate things about Children's Hospital—how it handles child abuse cases, for example —that legal entanglements would have prevented had I been naming names. One specific disclaimer: The Michael Jackson in this book is an amalgam of several patients, one of whom had another famous name. There are a lot of Michael Jacksons, though, and some of them have been patients at Children's Hospital. Mine is not one of those patients. Nevertheless, I offer the book as nonfiction, as the brief history of a new medical discipline, and as a practical guide to people in other cities who may conclude, after reading the tales that follow, that their town, too, needs a Children's Trauma Service.

IN THE BLINK OF AN EYE

One _____

The code room at Children's Hospital National Medical Center in Washington, D.C., is only a short distance from the helipad, but the three scrub-suited figures pull the gurney along at a dead run, green gowns billowing behind them. Seconds are precious when a child is hurt. The State Police helicopter medic jogs behind the gurney, service revolver bouncing against his brown flight suit.

On the gurney, a small boy struggles against the web straps that hold him tightly against a plywood backboard. Above the pink plastic collar that holds his neck immobile, his lips work frantically, but the whirring helicopter blades drown out his words until the stretcher is inside the hospital building, rolling toward the waiting trauma bay. The nurse nearest the boy's head bends close to his ear. "Tell me again, honey," she says. "I couldn't hear you before."

The voice is high and tremulous. "I said don't gimme no shots," the boy says loudly. "I can't *staaand* no shots!" The plea echoes off the textured walls as the gurney rolls into the code room and stops alongside the examining table. On the wall behind the bed, a large clock reads 6:04. As six sets of hands lift backboard and boy onto the examining table, the State Police medic appears in the doorway.

"This is Michael," he announces to the room in general. "Michael fell off an awning over a porch and landed on concrete steps about twelve feet down. He had loss of consciousness that lasted four or five minutes. He can move all extremities. His pulse has been good at about one sixty, respiration twenty-plus, blood pressure one fifteen over seventy and rock solid. Michael appears to be a very lucky little boy."

"Not lucky," Michael pouts from the examining table. "Not lucky while you tie me up like this. Don't gimme no shots, now," he snaps, his voice rising as a scrub-suited resident begins swabbing the crook of his left arm with an icy alcohol pad. "I said don't gimme no shots!"

1

"Michael, I've got to take a blood sample," the resident says. "Otherwise we won't know if you're okay. This will sting just for a second."

"Nooo, nooo, please, please don't—!" The pleas turn to a scream as the resident expertly spears a vein with a large-bore needle. Michael is indeed a lucky little boy, the resident reflects. Kids have very small veins; sometimes it takes two or three tries to get a blood sample.

Once the needle is in place, the sting quickly subsides, as do Michael's cries. Sobs and moans emanate from the bed, punctuated by little shrieks as the nurse on his left side presses EKG leads onto his torso. On the bank of monitors behind the anesthesiologist, an orange line jumps wildly on a display monitor, then settles into a familiar heartbeat wave form. A digital readout beside the wave form says that Michael's heart rate is 135 beats per minute, normal for a frightened child. The nurse near the head of the bed on the left side continues talking to Michael as she wraps a blood-pressure cuff around his arm. "Michael, you're in the hospital, and we're going to take good care of you, but first we've got to check you out and make sure you're all okay. Can you help us do that?"

"Don't want no help," Michael says. "I want to go home. Tell me when I can go home."

"Not for a little while yet, Michael," the nurse says. She turns and looks at the helicopter medic, who still stands in the doorway. "Family?" she asks.

"Not while we were there," the medic says quietly. "Mom was out somewhere." The resident on the left side of the table, his four tubes of blood drawn, slips the needle out of Michael's arm so smoothly that the boy appears not to notice; his attention is distracted by the resident on the right side, who is swabbing Michael's other arm.

"No more shots," Michael demands, panic in his voice. "I can't take no more shots." He shrieks for several seconds as the IV needle enters his arm, then begins sobbing again. "Please, please, can I go home now?" he begs.

The right-side resident is unable to suppress a smile. "Michael, I promise you we will let you go home as soon as we know you're absolutely okay and there's nothing wrong with you. But that's going to take a little while. Can you put up with us for a little while longer?"

"No! I wanna go home now! I'm gonna tell my daddy!" The two

residents grin at each other across the bed. From their point of view, Michael is a wonderful patient. All trauma patients should be so communicative. It's the ones who don't cry that they worry about.

Traumatic injury, the leading killer of children in this country, is a simple, straightforward disease, as simple as ABC: airway, breathing, and circulation. If the airway—the pathway between the mouth and nose and the lungs—is blocked, a child will strangle in a very few minutes. So the first priority of the medic in the field, and the trauma team in the hospital, is to provide the patient with an unobstructed airway.

Next most important is breathing. If an injury—a crushed chest, say—interferes with a child's ability to breathe, the child will suffocate, even if the airway is fine. Airway and breathing, the doctors teach the paramedics, are crucial; without them, you might as well forget all the rest. Put a tube down the patient's windpipe if you must; breathe for him with machines or mouth to mouth if you must. If you don't the patient will never reach the hospital alive.

Michael's team of doctors and nurses takes fresh reassurance from every wail of complaint. As long as he can shout and cry, his airway and his breathing are fine, just fine.

The nurse near Michael's left shoulder inflates a blood-pressure cuff and applies a stethoscope to Michael's lower arm. "One ten over seventy," she calls to the nurse-in-charge, who stands in one corner of the code room, arranging a dozen different printed forms. There are four doctors, four nurses, and a respiratory therapist in the code room. Each has specific duties, and each has a specific place to stand. The nurse-in-charge, who in quieter moments supervises the emergency room nursing staff, is in charge of making sure the paperwork gets done. Now she positions a form labeled Chronological Event Sheet on a small countertop. She writes "110/70" and notes the time, 6:05 P.M. Michael has been in the code room exactly one minute. On the right side of the sheet, under Remarks, the nurse jots "A/O"— alert and oriented. She pauses briefly, then smiles and adds, "Wants to go home."

If Michael is very lucky indeed, he will be allowed to go home tomorrow morning. Children have a near-miraculous ability to survive falls; in many cases they turn out to have no serious injuries at all. But a twelve-foot fall onto concrete steps is no minor accident. The trauma team will stubbornly assume the worst until the examinations and tests prove them wrong. Michael's greatest bit of luck was that he was brought to one of the nation's finest pediatric trauma centers, a place so sophisticated that it serves as a national model for other pediatric trauma programs, a place where children with potentially fatal injuries survive more than 95 percent of the time.

This good fortune, at the moment, is lost on Michael.

"I wanna get up," Michael complains. "Why you keep me tied up like this?"

"We don't want you to move around yet, Michael," nurse-left says in smooth, soothing tones. "We want to take pictures of your back and your neck and make sure you're okay before we let you start moving around, okay?"

"Not okay," Michael says. "When can I go home?"

"Michael," resident-right says, "you can go home when we know you're okay. Do you hurt anywhere, Michael?"

"My stomach hurts," Michael says.

Immediately, resident-right begins probing the abdomen with his fingertips. "Where, Michael? Tell me where it hurts. Does it hurt there? There?"

"No," Michael answers. "NoooOOO!" he screams as he feels resident-left swab his left arm with alcohol. "No shots! No more shots! Please, no more." This time the sting of the needle produces more sobs than screams, but the sobs continue long after the second IV needle is securely taped into place. With two IV lines functioning, the trauma team is ready for nearly any crisis. Even if Michael is bleeding internally, the trauma team can replace his losses through the two lines. Nurse-left pumps up the blood-pressure cuff again, calls out "one fifteen over seventy." Then she hooks the cuff to an automatic monitor. The machine will inflate the cuff and read Michael's blood pressure every 120 seconds and will display the result as a digital readout. In the corner of the room, the nurse-in-charge writes down the numbers, followed by the time: 6:06 P.M. Two minutes into the admission. The nurse-in-charge makes a note that both IVs are in place.

Michael, regaining his composure, abandons begging and pleading in favor of direct threats. "If you don't let me out of here right now," he says fiercely, "I'm going to tell my daddy and he's going to beat you up."

"Michael, can you go to the bathroom for me?" nurse-right asks.

4

Having finished cutting away Michael's clothing, she now stands at the boy's groin, holding a plastic specimen cup. "Michael, can you pee for me?" Michael doesn't answer. "Michael, if you can't pee for me, we have to put in a tube. Can you try real hard, Michael?" No answer.

Nurse-right looks at resident-right, who nods toward the supply cabinet. "A number ten," the resident says. The nurse abandons the plastic cup, goes to the supply cabinet and takes out a medium-size pediatric Foley catheter. Meanwhile, the resident pulls an examination glove onto his right hand and breaks open a package of sterile lubricant. In a moment, nurse-right will put the Foley into Michael's bladder, but first the resident must satisfy himself that Michael's pelvis is not broken. With his left hand, he presses firmly on one hip, then the other. "Michael, does that hurt?" he asks. The question, he knows by now, is a formality. If it hurt, he is sure, Michael would already have let him know. Michael remains silent.

"Michael, I've got to check your bottom," the resident says. "You're gonna feel like you need to go to the bathroom. This won't take but a couple of seconds, okay?" Michael remains silent. The resident smears a dab of lubricant on a gloved finger, then reaches between the small legs and slides the finger into Michael's rectum. From inside, the resident can feel the entire pelvic floor with his fingertip. If it is smooth and firm all the way around, everything is fine. If he feels lumps or if the prostate gland isn't where it ought to be, Michael may have a torn or damaged urethra, and the resident will order X-rays before putting in a catheter. If he finds a ridge, or if something moves, or if Michael screams with pain, the pelvis is broken and Michael will spend a long evening with an orthopedic surgeon.

"Hey," Michael exclaims. *"Hey!* Stop that! What you—*Stop that! Hey! Hey!"* There is profound indignation in Michael's voice, but no pain. More good luck. "You let me up from here," Michael sobs as the resident withdraws his finger. "I'm gonna kill you."

"I wouldn't blame you a bit, Michael," the resident mutters under his breath. It is not his favorite part of the trauma protocol, either. He smears his gloved fingertip across a piece of treated paper, folds the paper and hands it to the nurse-in-charge, who labels it, then checks it for the presence of blood.

Having satisfied himself that Michael's pelvis is all in one piece, the resident discards the examination glove and steps back. At the resident's nod, nurse-right pulls on a pair of sterile surgical gloves. Nurse-left holds out a small bowl of cotton balls that have been soaked in dark brown antiseptic. Nurse-right takes one, swabs off the entire length of Michael's penis. She throws the cotton ball into a trash can, takes a second one and swabs the tip of the penis a second time. Michael adds a moan or two to his sobs, but says nothing. The nurse tears open the sterile catheter package and carefully removes the tube inside. The nurse dips the small end of the tube into sterile lubricant, then slides it into the tip of the urethra. The second nurse grabs the other end of the tube and connects it to a plastic bag. When the tip of the catheter enters Michael's bladder, the tube turns pale yellow as urine flows through it. Simultaneously, a cry comes from the head of the bed.

"I gotta go to the bathroom right *now!*" Michael wails. When the Foley dilates the tiny muscle that holds the bladder closed, it produces the same sensation as an urgent need to urinate.

"Don't worry about it, Michael," resident-right says. "We've got it under control. You just relax and let it go." The nurse and the resident examine the bag as urine begins to collect in it. It is pale and clear, with no sign of blood.

Michael continues to cry, and suddenly the resident becomes aware of a harsh scratchiness in the child's voice. Crying can produce the deep congestion the resident hears, but so can other things. Moving up to the head of the table, he listens intently to Michael's chest with his stethoscope. There are breath sounds on both sides, but something doesn't sound quite right. The resident moves the stethoscope disk from left side to right side, listening intently. The breath sounds from the left side are not as distinct as on the right.

"Michael," the resident says, his voice still friendly but with an added twinge of authority to it. "Tell me where it hurts, Michael." As he says the words, he reaches across the examining table and presses Michael's left shoulder with his fingertips. No response. He moves his fingers over the left nipple, presses. No response. Under the armpit; no response. Down the ribs . . .

Michael lets out a shrill, gurgling scream.

The resident withdraws his hand immediately. Michael stops screaming and begins crying again, but the resident remains tensely alert; this is no longer a routine admission.

"X-ray," he calls over his shoulder. "Ready for X-ray. Now." Then to resident-left, he adds "ABG. Stat."

An arterial blood gas sample is the surest way to tell how well Michael's lungs are functioning. It is also the most painful of all the procedures the trauma team performs. Often the team will put off this procedure as long as possible, and on occasion the patient is doing so obviously well that they can forgo the test altogether. But not this time. While the X-ray technician wheels her lumbering portable machine into the trauma bay, resident-left quickly swabs off the inside of Michael's left wrist. The medications nurse hands him a special needle that has a thin flexible tube attached to the blunt end. Taking careful aim, the resident plunges the needle deep into Michael's wrist, searching for the radial artery.

The scream that results is even more worrisome than before. It is a long, liquid cry that ends with a gasp, then a cough, then several short cries as resident-left moves the needle back and forth, hunting blindly for the artery. Suddenly the thin tube turns bright red. Resident-left holds the needle perfectly still while the medications nurse lets the bright arterial blood flow into a small tube. "Okay," she says, and resident-left removes the needle with a rapid jerk. He hands the wrist over to nurse-left, who presses a sterile dressing against the puncture site and holds it there. The medications nurse hands the tube of blood to the nurse-in-charge, who slaps a label around the tube, plunges it into a plastic cup filled with ice, and walks to the door of the code room. "Blood gas," she calls, and a waiting lab technician trots over, takes the plastic cup from her, and lopes off down the hallway.

"Chest first," resident-right instructs the X-ray technician. Ordinarily, the first X-ray is taken of the neck, but resident-right isn't worried about Michael's neck. The cervical collar is still in place, adding to Michael's unhappiness, but it will keep. Michael also has a growing lump on his forehead, but that, too, can wait. Right now, the resident is keenly interested in Michael's chest. While resident-left, nurse-left, nurse-right, and the X-ray technician are busy sliding an X-ray plate under the backboard, resident-right moves back to the boy's side.

"Michael," he says sharply, grasping the boy's right hand. "Squeeze my fingers, Michael. Good. Now can you wiggle your toes for me?" Michael bangs his heels on the backboard. "Good. Michael, we're going to take a picture of your chest now. We're all going out of the room for just a second, but we'll be right back, okay?"

7

"You can stay gone," Michael replies wearily. "I don't like you."

The nine trauma team members duck out the two doorways of the code room as the X-ray tech, wearing a lead apron, makes the final adjustments to her machine. "Shooting," she calls out.

"Don't shoot," Michael wails. "Don't shoot me no more."

The X-ray machine whirs, then clicks. "Okay," the technician calls. Two nurses and a resident help remove the X-ray plate, and the tech hands it to an orderly standing just outside the doorway. The orderly heads for the elevators.

The standard admission X-ray sequence is neck, chest, pelvis. Her routine disrupted, the tech decides to do the pelvis next. This time, she calls out "X-ray" instead of "shooting," and Michael remains calm.

For the neck X-ray, nurse-left puts on a lead apron and lead gloves. The X-ray technician positions the machine's lens next to the right side of Michael's neck. Nurse-left holds the X-ray plate vertically on the other side of the neck. "Ready?" the X-ray tech asks.

"No," Michael responds. "Not ready. Never ready." Grinning, the X-ray technician manipulates her controls. Another whir, click, and she calls out, "All done."

Resident-right wastes no time getting back to Michael's side, though now he stands on the left side, next to resident-left, listening again to Michael's chest with his stethoscope. "Don't open it yet," he calls across the examining table to nurse-right, "because I want to see the chest X-ray first, but make sure the thoracotomy tray is handy, willya?"

Outside the code room, a wall phone rings, and the evening-shift nursing supervisor picks it up, listens a moment, then begins to jot numbers on a pad. She hangs up the phone, turns around and repeats the numbers aloud to resident-right. His reply is not to the nursing supervisor but to nurse-right: "Okay, open the tray and get it set up. But I still want to look at the X-ray. Where's the X-ray?"

As if in answer to his question, the white-coated orderly strides into the room, and snaps an X-ray film into a light box. The two residents quickly walk around the examining table and stand in front of the light box, talking in low tones and pointing to a shadow on the left side of Michael's chest. After a few moments, they walk back to Michael's left side. The thoracotomy tray, containing a chest tube and the tools necessary to implant it, lies open on a small stainless steel table. Nurse-left has already removed the web strap that kept Michael's arms from thrashing around. Now she holds the boy's left arm so that his side is exposed and accessible.

Resident-right pulls on surgical gloves, and begins to bathe Michael's ribs with brown antiseptic liquid. Michael flinches at the resident's touch and moans. The resident says, "Michael, I've got to work on your side for a minute here. I'm going to put some medicine in your side now. It's going to sting for just a minute, okay?"

"Lemme alone," Michael says quietly. "I can't breathe. Lemme alone."

"I know you can't breathe, Michael," the resident says. "That's what I've got to fix." The nurse hands him a syringe filled with lidocaine, a local anesthetic. With a gloved finger, the resident counts down Michael's rib cage, one, two, three, four . . . he inserts the needle between the fourth and fifth ribs and pushes the plunger on the syringe, moving the needle as he squeezes, distributing the painkiller under Michael's skin. Michael manages a gargle, followed by a cough; a collapsed lung makes it difficult to yell. That was what had initially tipped off the resident. You don't worry about the ones who cry and scream; you worry about the ones who become quiet.

Resident-right tests the anesthetic by pushing a finger against the rib he now knows is broken. Michael stays quiet. Good. The pain block is in place. Now for the chest tube . . .

The resident swabs the skin once more with antiseptic, then takes a scalpel and makes a small incision, half an inch long, between the fourth and fifth ribs. Michael doesn't flinch or cry out. Working quickly, the resident deepens the incision until he can see the bluish membrane that surrounds the lungs. He slips a gloved finger into the incision, which keeps it open and also keeps it from bleeding. A nurse takes the scalpel from his outstretched hand, and holds an opened sterile package toward him. He twists his head to look at the package. "No, that's not big enough," he says. "Gimme a twenty-four." The nurse turns to a supply rack, grabs another sterile package, tears it open and holds the package out. "Perfect," the resident says, lifting the tube out of the sterile pack.

On one end of the clear plastic tube there are pale blue rings, exactly one centimeter apart. The resident begins to thread this end of the

9

tube past his finger and into the surgical wound. When the tube is about a centimeter deep, he removes his finger; the cut immediately closes around the tubing, and the resident grips the tube tightly as he continues pushing it into Michael's chest. The nurse holds the other, nonsterile end of the tubing. "Hook that up to about twenty centimeters, wouldja?" the resident says. The amount of suction necessary to support a column of water twenty centimeters high will be just right to restore the natural vacuum to Michael's chest cavity and cause his lung to reinflate. Now the resident has to find the air pocket left by the collapsing lung. After it enters Michael's side, the flexible plastic tube slides along between the chest wall and the pleural membrane. The resident continues pushing the tube in, three centimeters, four— until suddenly, large pink bubbles begin to race down the tube. Air, and only a little bit of blood. Michael, the resident reflects once again, is a very lucky little boy.

The resident glances at the wall clock. It is 6:18 P.M., fourteen minutes since Michael rolled in the door. Not bad, not bad at all. It is not the resident's record for completing a trauma protocol, but on the other hand he doesn't see a pneumothorax that often. Children's ribs are pliable; usually they bend without breaking. It takes a special impact, like the edge of a concrete step after a twelve-foot fall, to break a rib and drive it into a lung.

Now the resident's attention moves to Michael's forehead, which continues to swell. From the shape of the lump, the resident can see that Michael must have been looking down when he hit; the left side is badly swollen, but the right side is enlarged, too. This presents a fresh problem: The last item on the resident's trauma checklist is a nasogastric tube, the tube that enters the nose on its way to the stomach. Trauma patients sometimes become nauseous, so it is a routine precaution to empty the stomach.

On the other hand, if Michael's head injury includes damage to any of the sinus cavities behind his nose, the nasogastric tube, instead of curving around toward the esophagus, could simply penetrate straight through the sinuses and come dangerously close to Michael's brain. It is a tough call to make; should he attempt to put in the NG tube or not?

The decision is interrupted by the arrival of Michael's other two X-rays. Resident-right and resident-left go immediately to the film of

Michael's neck. Resident-left points with a ballpoint pen to the atlas, the first bone of the spine, the one that attaches to the base of the skull. In medical shorthand, that is C-1, the first cervical vertebra. Resident-left counts downward, one, two, three, four, five, six, seven. Then resident-right does the same thing. Michael's neck is fine. They both saw all seven neck bones. It's when you can't see one that you worry. "C-spine's clear," resident-right announces. Immediately, nurse-left begins unbuckling the pink plastic collar that has held Michael's neck immobile ever since the ambulance crew arrived at the accident scene. Michael lets out a long sigh as he experimentally moves his head from side to side. The straps that hold him to the backboard stay in place; a child so anxious to go home makes the nurses cautious. If Michael were completely unrestrained, he might abruptly try to leave. He would not get far with two IVs, a chest tube, and a Foley catheter in place, but he might hurt himself trying. When the nurses are sure Michael is calm, the last of the straps will come off.

Meanwhile, the two residents finish their examination of the X-rays and return to their positions on both sides of the examining table. Resident-right has made his decision: The NG tube can wait. "I want CAT scans of his head and abdomen before we do anything else," the resident says.

There is a bustle of activity as the trauma team prepares to move the patient to the CAT scanner on the second floor. Outside the doorway, the assistant director of nursing punches a number into a wall phone, pauses briefly, then announces, "We're on our way up," into the receiver. Inside the code room, nurses and residents begin rearranging tubing, moving intravenous fluid bags, attaching the EKG leads to a battery-powered portable monitor. The nurse-in-charge reaches into a manila envelope and withdraws a wristband, already stamped "Acute Patient #10664, Dr. Eichelberger." She picks up a pen, then pauses. "Michael," she calls out, walking to the bedside, "Michael, what's your last name?"

"Jackson," the boy replies.

"Get outta here," the nurse-in-charge snorts. "Don't you think I know who Michael Jackson is?"

For the first time since he came in the door, Michael giggles. "Not *that* Michael Jackson," he says, "but my name's Michael Jackson, too."

11

"I don't believe that for one minute," the nurse says, which draws another giggle. Already, she is writing "Jackson, Michael," on the wristband. She slips the band onto Michael's left wrist, then returns to her stack of forms and begins filling Michael's name in all the spaces stamped "Acute patient #10664, Dr. Eichelberger."

Two _____

Marty Eichelberger fought the hook for years before he gave in and admitted that treating children was what he liked best. It makes a better story to blame the decision on his mentor, Dr. C. Everett Koop, and that is the story he most often tells, but if you press him, Dr. Eichelberger will admit that ultimately his wife, Nancy, made the choice for him.

Marty had always thought of himself as a family man. He grew up in a close-knit family, and it seemed only natural to start a family of his own. Nancy agreed, and Todd Eichelberger was born midway through his father's residency; Lindsay Eichelberger arrived during the last year of Marty's residency.

Those were tough times, as all residencies are. When Marty came home at all, he came home bone tired, sometimes irritable, always full of stories about this patient or that doctor or the latest political squabble or rumor of intrigue around the hospital. Talking helped Marty loosen the tensions that built up inside him, and Nancy was always a good, thoughtful listener.

When he had rotated through cardiology in medical school, his hours suddenly improved. Cardiologists worked gentlemen's hours; it was the heart surgeons who had to watch their patients round the clock. Cardiologists referred people to heart surgeons. Marty cherished the extra time he got to spend with Nancy and the kids and made up his mind to be a cardiologist.

Then his cardiology rotation had ended, and he found himself in the pediatric surgery service at Philadelphia Children's Hospital, working under Dr. Koop. Best known to the lay public as the current surgeon general of the United States, within the medical profession Dr. Koop is considered one of the finest pediatric surgeons in America.

Under Dr. Koop, Marty Eichelberger discovered that he had a

13

Alan Doelp

surgeon's hands. He could open a kid up, find his way through the tiny anatomy, make the necessary repairs, and be talking to the kid that afternoon. Cardiology was fine, and the hours were great, but this was real gratification. Though Marty came home late and tired, the stories he brought with him were grand heroic tales of ills cured and lives saved. If Dr. Koop was the consummate teacher, Marty Eichelberger was the ideal student: quick, bright, and energetic. Together the two men worked near-miracles every day.

Marty knew now that he would be a surgeon, and as soon as he was graduated from medical school, he began a general surgery residency at Case Western Reserve University, in Cleveland. However, it still remained for him to choose a specialty. He was torn; Dr. Koop had shown him all the wonders of pediatric surgery, but he fretted at spending all his nights with other people's children instead of his own. Orthopedics would be better, he thought: Orthopods worked hard, but the hours were better, the on-call schedules less grueling. During his residency, he spent his two years of military service doing orthopedic surgery at the Naval Academy.

After his Navy tour, Dr. Eichelberger returned to Case Western, and began to plan a career as an orthopedic surgeon. He shopped for jobs, and found one at Case. He had begun to make the arrangements when his wife stopped him. "This is crazy," she said. "You don't want to be an orthopod. You want to be a pediatric surgeon."

Years after that conversation, the memory is still fresh in Dr. Eichelberger's mind. "I said, 'What do you mean?' and she said, 'You've known all along that this is what you want to do. If you go into orthopedics just because the call schedule's easier, you'll hate yourself for it.' "

The next day, Dr. Eichelberger made two phone calls. The first was to Case. The second was to Dr. Koop.

The following July, Dr. Eichelberger moved his family to Philadelphia, and for the next two years they didn't see much of him. The fraternity of pediatric surgeons is a small one, and no newcomers enter without first serving a two-year postgraduate fellowship in pediatric surgery. In a sense it is like an extra residency, two more years tacked onto the five years of surgical residency that follow the four years of medical school. By the time Marty finished his two-year hitch under Dr. Koop, he would have invested thirteen years of his life in becoming a pediatric surgeon.

In Marty's view, it was a fair trade. Not only does he get to do what he most enjoys, which is healing sick kids, he also has the satisfaction of knowing that the Washington, D.C., area is, statistically, one of the safest parts of the country for Todd and Lindsay Eichelberger to grow up in.

Twenty years ago, R. Adams Cowley, the patron saint of trauma medicine, rocked the medical establishment with his oft-repeated remark that "you live or die depending on where you have your accident, because they take you to the nearest hospital." Trauma victims, Dr. Cowley said, were getting second-rate care, and because of that, some of them were dying unnecessarily.

Ten years ago, when he realized that pediatric trauma cases were different from adult cases—so different that children were dying unnecessarily—Marty Eichelberger started making a few waves of his own.

Dr. Eichelberger cites the spleen as an example. In an injured adult, it is commonplace to remove the spleen if it is bleeding. An adult will probably never miss the organ. But in a child, the spleen is vitally important to the development of an immune system. Remove an injured child's spleen, and the child will recover, go home, and appear to be completely normal until months or even years later, when the child catches a cold and dies without warning. A good pediatric trauma surgeon, then, knows he must, if possible, repair the spleen, not remove it.

During his two-year hitch at Philadelphia Children's Hospital, Dr. Eichelberger spent precious spare time browsing through the medical literature and found example after example of profound differences between adult and pediatric trauma. The information was all there, but nobody had ever gathered it all together. Dr. Eichelberger did and, armed with his sheaf of reprints, he began to proselytize among his colleagues.

It is hard to ignore a man with a stack of journal articles in his hand and the gleam of revelation in his eye. Soon, Philadelphia Children's Hospital had a trauma service, and young Dr. Eichelberger was in charge of it.

And his patients did better. There was no magic about it; Dr. Eichelberger had made no new medical discoveries. He had simply begun to apply state-of-the-art medicine in a systematic, methodical fashion. The only remarkable thing was nobody had done it before.

Three _____

Mirean Coleman watched the stretcher roll past her and into the code room. She smiled at little Michael's running commentary and winced when he cried out. She watched carefully, straining to hear what she could of the conversation inside the code room. She did not step inside.

Mirean carries one of the bright red pagers that identify members of the trauma stat team, but she is neither a physician nor a nurse. Mirean is a social worker; her job is to admit the patient's family to the hospital.

In pediatric trauma, Marty Eichelberger preaches, you don't just have an injured child, you have an injured family. Trauma team members repeat that rule so often and with such conviction that one would think they had invented it, but they did not. The principle that child and family should be treated as one is not new at Children's Hospital; it was firmly in place long before Dr. Eichelberger arrived.

To this day there are hospitals that routinely separate children from their parents for at least part of the hospital day. The justifications for this practice are at best vague, usually couched in haughty and unintelligible medical jargon that attempts to convey the message that it is best for the child. Nothing could be farther from the truth. In overwhelming numbers, children whose parents stay with them behave better, tolerate procedures better, and recover from their illnesses faster than children left to convalesce alone.

The staff at Children's Hospital National Medical Center knew this intuitively long before the statistics proved it. At Children's Hospital, there are two beds in every room; a hospital bed for the patient and a sofa bed for a parent. At Children's Hospital parents are not only allowed, they are strongly encouraged to stay with their kids.

When a child is injured, family relationships are traumatized along with the patient. For the child, getting hurt translates to getting

16

caught doing something dangerous. He is used to being scolded or even punished for doing dangerous things; now he knows he's done something *really* bad, and the fear of imagined punishment blends with the pain of the injuries to create a living nightmare. Often, the nightmare revisits the child afterward, at night, for months or years.

In the experience of the children's trauma team, a calm, loving, supportive family can blunt the terror and lessen the nightmares. But it is tough to be calm at such a time. Parents are accustomed to having absolute control of, and complete responsibility for, their child. Now, suddenly, the child belongs not to them but to a gang of strangers in sterile pajamas in a distant examining room. In an instant, everything normal in life has vanished, leaving only disorientation and chaos. Some parents simply go numb. A few panic and fight with the hospital staff; most merely fight with each other.

Medical people have known for generations that traumatic injury produces family stresses; Children's Hospital is one of the few that does anything about it.

When the helicopter medic turned to leave the code room, Mirean stopped him. "Anything on the family?" she asked.

The medic frowned. "Not a lot," he said. "A neighbor called the ambulance. There was one younger child in the apartment, but mom wasn't there. Nobody knew where she was. Her name is . . ." he consulted his papers ". . . Sarah. I don't have a last name. She just moved there a few weeks ago, apparently."

"Okay, thanks," Mirean replied. "I'll watch for her." She turned and walked down the hallway, to the emergency room main desk. Behind the desk, in a cramped room, is the trauma service's communications center. "We don't have a family yet," she said to the operator seated inside. "Can you find out from the ambulance people whether they ever notified anyone?"

"Sure," the operator said. "Got any names?"

"The patient's name is Michael," Mirean said. "The mother's name, I think, is Sarah. No last names yet." She repeated the address where the accident happened, an apartment complex in the Maryland suburbs. "The neighbors didn't know where mom was."

"No problem," the operator said, picking up a phone. Mirean left and walked back to her station just outside the code room.

In minutes, the comm operator joined her. "Mom was apparently in the laundry room. Her name is Sarena Jackson. She's on her way.

And," he said, "there is a gentleman at the desk who says he's the father. Want to come see him?"

Mirean Coleman moves and talks with a practiced slowness that affects everyone around her. She fairly radiates tranquillity; just chatting with her is a relaxing experience. Her ability to soothe and calm is almost hypnotic; it is difficult to be frantic in her presence.

Michael's father, a burly man in expensive-looking casual clothes, was busy being frantic. As Mirean rounded the corner the man was pacing up and down in front of the nursing station, flexing his shoulders, taking deep breaths, and banging a fist into the palm of his hand. Mirean caught his eye and smiled as she walked toward him. The man did not return the smile; he strode toward her rapidly, almost menacingly. "Where is he?" the man demanded, interrupting Mirean as she introduced herself.

Mirean let her smile diminish a trace. "Michael is in with the doctors right now," she said. The man opened his mouth to speak, but Mirean continued. "He's awake and talking to them, but it'll be a few minutes before we can go see him," she said, anticipating the next question. "While we're waiting, it would be very helpful to the doctors to have some more information about Michael. Does he have a regular pediatrician?"

"Yes, he does," the man answered. He mentioned a name, and an address in the District of Columbia. Mirean dutifully noted it on the form she carried, then paused.

"Why don't we go down to my office?" she suggested. "We can sit down. Is Michael taking any drugs or medicines that you know of?" She moved gracefully down the hall, away from the code room, the father safely in tow. Some social workers hate the emergency room because it is always full of frantic parents. Mirean thrives there. The parents aren't hostile, she says, they're just anxious and they want to help. Give them some way to help, some way to feel just a little bit like they're in control, and they always relax.

Mirean's office was once an examining room. With a desk, a sofa, a chair, and a file cabinet in the room, there is scarcely any space left to move around inside. The sofa partially blocks the door, and Mirean and Michael's father had to squeeze in single file. Mirean sat down at the desk, pen poised over her admission form. "Does Michael have any existing medical problems?" she asked.

"No."

"Is he allergic to any drugs or foods?"

"Not that I know of."

"Does he take any medications regularly?"

"No."

"Do you know if he's had a tetanus shot recently?"

"No, I don't know. His mother would know."

"How old is Michael?"

"Seven. Seven and a half."

"What's his birthday?"

"Eighth of July."

"Has he ever been in the hospital before?"

"No. Except when he was born, that is."

Mirean continued to write on the admission form for a moment, then looked up. "I'm sorry, I don't even know your name."

"Jackson," the father replied. "Kenneth R. Jackson."

Mirean wrote in the name, then stood up. "Let me go give this information to the doctors and see if I can find out how Michael's doing now. Can I bring you a cup of coffee?" The father shook his head. "Okay," she continued. "I'll be back in a few minutes."

In the code room, the surgical resident was in the midst of inserting the chest tube in Michael's side. Mirean stuck her head in the door and caught the eye of the nurse-in-charge. "The father's here," Mirean said quietly. "The mother's supposed to be here any minute. Anything I can tell them?"

The nurse-in-charge consulted her chronological event sheet. "He's been stable the whole time. Alert and oriented. Moves all extremities. He has a left pneumothorax resulting from a fifth-rib fracture and a nasty lump on his forehead, but he's neurologically okay. You heard him carrying on?" Mirean grinned, nodded.

The surgical resident looked up. "Tell them Michael's a very lucky little boy. I'll come talk to them in a few minutes."

"Okay, thanks." Mirean turned and walked down the hallway, around the nursing station, then back up a second hallway parallel to the first, tracing an elongated horseshoe path to get to her office at the end of the hall. Mirean's office is deliberately distant from the code room; in those first few breathless minutes after a hurt child arrives, there is no thought given to painkillers. It is the single cold-blooded reality of an otherwise compassionate enterprise. A crying child is a child very much alive; the trauma team takes fresh reassurance from every shriek.

Parents, in their anxiety, seldom understand this. To them, their child's cries are an almost irresistible summons to help. So Mirean's office is conveniently out of earshot. If a parent were allowed in the code room, the trauma team might spend precious seconds on explanations or courtesy. Until the trauma team declares a patient stable, no one, not even another physician, enters the code room uninvited. Ultimately, trauma is a surgical disease; the code room is a place where surgical priorities prevail. It is, like the operating suite upstairs, one of the few places where parents cannot go.

One of Mirean Coleman's principal duties is to see that child and parents are reunited at the earliest possible moment. Meanwhile, she shuttles back and forth between parents and code room, relaying information. "The surgeon says Michael is a very lucky little boy," Mirean said as she squeezed through the narrow doorway.

"Is he going to be all right?"

Mirean answered the question carefully. "They're still doing their examination," she said, "but they say he's been stable and alert the whole time. The major thing they've found is a broken rib, which caused one of his lungs to partially collapse. They put a tube in his side, and that will allow the lung to reinflate." She allowed her smile to widen. "The most important thing is that he has been alert and talking to us the whole time, which means his brain is okay. He can move both arms and both legs, so we know he's not paralyzed. He's got quite a bump on his head, but it doesn't seem to bother him. Right now they're making sure he doesn't have any internal injuries." Mirean paused. "And he is very, very upset with us because we stuck him with needles. He really didn't like that at all."

Mr. Jackson smiled for the first time. "I know. We practically have to tie him down to take him to the doctor."

"In just a few minutes we can go see him," Mirean said. She was about to continue when someone knocked, then pushed the door open. It was the emergency room desk clerk.

"Hi, Mirean," the clerk said. "Mrs. Jackson's here." The clerk backed away from the narrow doorway, turned. "Go on in," she said. A tall, heavyset woman wearing wrinkled gray slacks and a flower-print cotton blouse appeared in the doorway.

"Hi. I'm Mirean Coleman. Come on in," Mirean said as the woman turned sideways to squeeze in the door, which blocked her view of the room until she was inside. Then Mrs. Jackson caught sight of Mr. Jackson, who meanwhile had stood up. Their eyes met, locked briefly. There was no compassion in either gaze.

"What happened? How did this happen?" Mr. Jackson demanded, his tone accusing.

"You know exactly how it happened," she replied. "He's gone out on that awning before, and I asked you to put a lock on that window so he couldn't open it. That stick you put in the window didn't stop him; he climbed up on a chair and took it out."

"And where were you while all this was happening?"

Mrs. Jackson's gaze grew more hostile. "I was in the laundry room," she said, "which as you know is on the other end of the building, in the basement. Because I thought he was safe!"

Mirean decided it was time to intervene. "Mrs. Jackson, I just came from talking to the doctors, and they said they have everything under control right now. They said he was very lucky." She looked slowly from one parent to the other. "Why don't we all sit down?" she suggested. "I need to explain a couple of things.

"The first thing is that Michael is a very frightened little boy, and he's going to need reassurance and support from both of you. He does have some injuries and we know he's going to be in the hospital at least for tonight and possibly longer than that. He'll be sleeping in a strange place, full of strange people who give him shots. The only familiar thing he has to hold on to is you two.

"Children are a lot more perceptive than we give them credit for sometimes," she continued. "If there is tension between you two, Michael is going to pick that up, and he's going to think it's his fault. That's not going to be good for Michael. He'll recover a lot quicker, and have fewer problems, if you're there to help him."

She looked back and forth from one parent to the other. "Whatever your differences are, and it's none of my business, I would hope you could put them aside for Michael's sake. If you feel you can't do that, then it would probably be best for you to visit him separately instead of together."

Mirean paused, let the silence grow for several seconds. The Jacksons looked at each other, at Mirean, and back at each other. Finally, Mirean spoke again.

"Let me go see if they're ready to let us visit with Michael," she said, standing up. "Do you need to make any phone calls?" She gestured at the phone on her desk. "Dial nine first. We also have WATS lines if you need to call anyone out of town."

At the code room, Mirean discovered that Michael was being readied for the trip to X-ray. "Hold off for a minute," she told the nurse-in-charge. "Let me get the parents over here."

She tapped on her own office door before she walked in. Mr. and Mrs. Jackson were sitting together on the couch. Mrs. Jackson was dabbing at a tear. "They're getting ready to take him to X-ray," Mirean said. "If we hurry, we can go see him right now." She didn't ask whether they wanted to go together or separately; they clearly had already decided.

Four

The eyewitnesses differed on exactly how far little David Myers flew through the air after the car hit him, but their consensus was about fifty feet, so the police wrote "50 ft." on their report. When David's father, David Senior, paced off the distance later, he put it closer to one hundred feet. But that was later, and the difference was, as they say, a lawyer's difference. When the car hit little David, he sailed through the air like a forty-pound rag doll, rolled once when he landed, and came to rest on his side, curled up in an almost fetal position in the street, his eyes wide and unblinking, his legs bent at impossible angles, unmoving, unconscious, dying.

David's father came charging out the front door of their apartment, running like a madman. He was the first person to reach little David. The driver sat, frozen, inside his car. Traffic began to pile up on Alabama Avenue as people left their cars to get a better look. People came out of other apartments and clustered around.

David Senior knelt beside his son, his mind ablaze yet somehow almost numb. He moved with unaccustomed slowness to touch little David's forehead, testing to see if it still felt firm and warm. He moved his finger down and gently touched one eyelid. The eye didn't move; the pupil was wide and did not shrink in the bright Sunday sunshine.

The boy took a breath, and it was the long, shuddering, almost gasping kind of breath that you hear when a child has been crying. A froth of pink appeared at little David's lips.

"We called nine-one-one," somebody in the crowd said. "They said they'd send an ambulance."

David Senior's mind was a fog, paralyzed and panicky at the same time, but he heard the word *ambulance*. He moved to cradle little David in his arms, then drew back, afraid to touch anything. He spoke loudly but without looking up: "Call them back," he said, "and tell them please to hurry."

◆ ◆ ◆

Whenever they discussed it afterward, David's parents always looked for something, even a little thing, to be grateful for. They agreed they should be grateful, very grateful that they had put up the Christmas tree the night before. Little David had relished every minute of it, and they had been forced to do most of the work late Saturday night, after their son was in bed and couldn't help.

Christmas, to a four-year-old, is a magical time. Presents need only be wished for and they will appear under that wonderful tree on Christmas morning. David was old enough to remember the previous Christmas, young enough not to understand that only a limited number of presents can fit under the tree. On several occasions, he had hauled out the Sears catalog and gone through the toy section with a pencil, marking the things he wanted. He had already marked nearly everything and had begun refining his choices, which at the time centered around the action-adventure toys known as Thundercats.

The religious significance of Christmas was lost on David, but his parents were determined to change that; as soon as he was old enough to be shushed, his parents had begun to take him to Sunday services at a nearby Baptist church, where lately he had remained reasonably quiet, though he squirmed and fidgeted a great deal. Earlier that morning, they had pried him away from the Christmas tree, and his mother had lectured him in the car on the way to church. "You got to sit still and be quiet and listen to the man talk about Jesus," she said sternly.

Little David was in no mood for sternness; Christmas was too near. "Listen to the man talk about Jesus," he repeated slowly, getting the sound of it. Then he pointed an accusing finger at his mother. "You," he said, "got to sit still and be quiet and listen to the man talk about Jesus!" Both parents grinned at each other; there was no denying he was a sharp kid. With that kind of energy and that kind of quick, bright mind, there would be no stopping him. The savings account earmarked for his college education was already substantial; Patricia and David Myers had vowed that their only child would have every opportunity.

In church, little David made a valiant effort to listen to the man talk about Jesus, but Baptist sermons tend to run long, and before the service was over, little David was fidgeting so energetically that his father finally whisked him outside, lectured him sternly for a few seconds, then let him run around to work off the excess steam. Little David seemed to have boundless energy, so much energy that once they had taken him to a doctor, who had diagnosed him as hyperactive. Mom worried about the diagnosis, but dad dismissed it as nonsense. After all, he himself was full of compulsive energy; the boy just took after his father, that was all. A boy with lots of energy would achieve more. The last thing he needed was drugs to take away all his energy.

On the way home from church, they stopped at the Sears store to look at video recorders. Life had been good to them; Pat worked at FBI headquarters, David Senior at the National Weather Service. With the income from two good, secure government jobs, they had been able to save a great deal of money toward—whatever. Little David's college, vacations at Disney World, trips home to Brunswick, Georgia, a house in the suburbs . . .

They had decided to buy a VCR to give to Pat's mother for Christmas. Eventually, they would buy a video camera so they could make recordings on their own VCR of little David, and some day, when the boy was grown and off on his own, they'd be able to pop a tape in the machine and remember this golden time. David was an exceptionally handsome boy, even if they did say so themselves—which they often did—and they carried photographs around to prove it. Home video movies would be even better; a VCR for Grandma was an essential first step.

Little David, seeing the Sears catalog come to life, ran off to the toy department to make an advance withdrawal against Christmas Day. His mother took off in pursuit, while dad stayed near the TV section. The Redskins game was in full swing, and as halftime approached, the Skins pushed downfield and scored a tying touchdown. The television crowds cheered, and David Senior stayed glued to the set until Mom returned with little David in tow. The Giants blasted ahead to a first down, and the announcer reminded viewers that "this half isn't over yet." Reluctantly, David Senior moved away from the televisions toward the exit; the two-minute warning had just sounded.

The family car had a radio, but David Senior didn't turn it on to follow the game. He had a thing about car radios, thought they distracted his driving. He was as meticulous about his driving as he had always been about his weather maps, and being so good with weather maps is what had got him promoted to a supervisory job at the weather service. He turned onto Alabama Avenue, found a parking spot on the street almost directly across from the apartment.

David Senior took David Junior's hand as they dashed across the street toward the apartment. The standing rule was that little David never crossed the street alone, but against the day when the boy would be allowed out on his own, David Senior, as he always did, made an exaggerated business of checking to his left, then to his right. Cars driving down the straight stretch of Alabama Avenue that runs alongside St. Elizabeth's Hospital tended to ignore the thirty-mile-per-hour speed limit; sometimes they drove by so fast it even scared the grown-ups. Now the street was clear, and father and son headed for the apartment.

Mom, as she often did, hung back. There were old boxes and papers in the car, and she carefully gathered them up and squeezed everything together in a bundle she could take directly around to the trash dumpster in back of the apartment building. In her mind there was nothing worse than a junky car. The two Davids, who both acted as if they were always in a hurry, had long since gotten out of the habit of waiting around for Mom. It was almost a family tradition; David Senior and David Junior would open the apartment door, and little David would greet Mom a few seconds later when she walked in.

The Christmas tree was just inside the door, and David Senior stopped long enough to switch on the lights before heading upstairs, where he turned on the television set and tuned in the Redskins game. The second half was about to start. Had they made the touchdown? He kept his eyes glued to the screen, waiting for the score to be shown. It was as though the TV producers knew he was waiting; they ran a commercial, then another commercial, but no score. David Senior kept his eyes locked on the television.

"Where Mommy?" little David asked. When Dad didn't reply, he asked it again, louder. "Where Mommy?"

"Mommy's downstairs," Dad replied distractedly. He hadn't heard her key in the lock, but it had been long enough; if she wasn't downstairs, she would be any second. David bolted down the stairs. A few seconds later, Dad heard the door open. Good, he thought. There's Mommy. He sat down to continue watching the game.

◆ ◆ ◆

One eyewitness said that when little David ran to the curb of the forbidden street, he stopped and carefully looked both ways before he ran across. He ran to the other side and down the sidewalk to the family car. He looked inside the car and tried to open the passenger-side door, then ran around behind the car. According to the witness, he again looked both ways before he dashed into the street, but parked just behind the Myers's car was a large van, which partially blocked his view. Little David apparently never saw or heard the approaching Buick Riviera.

◆ ◆ ◆

Patricia Myers took her time straightening things in the car, then crossed the street and headed toward the bank of trash dumpsters behind the apartment building. There was no need to hurry; church was over, it was a comfortably crisp Sunday afternoon, and she knew David Senior would be tied up with the football game for another hour or two. Perhaps she would curl up in a chair with a book, or perhaps get out her Bible and read more about the Apostle Paul's ministry to the Romans, which is what the sermon that morning had been about. But certainly, there was no cause to hurry.

She was just rounding the corner of the apartment building when she heard the squeal of tires. No cause for alarm: You heard squealing tires all the time around here. People drove like maniacs down Alabama Avenue sometimes. It was not, she thought again, a proper place to raise a boy. They ought to have a place out in the suburbs, a proper house with a yard, on a quiet street. She had suggested it many times, but David Senior had resisted. "When we get some more money saved up," he would always say. Pat thought that was non-sense; they had plenty of savings, more than enough for a down payment. But David was stubborn. "We can't spend all that money. What if we suddenly needed it for something?"

She saw the Buick's red taillights, and still nothing registered. Then down the street, she saw a small, still form, and she gasped and thought, Oh my God, there's been a child hit, but still it didn't register. Then she heard her husband shout, "David! David!" and she saw him running toward the street, and suddenly she knew that the body in the street was her own child, and she began to run, faster and faster, toward the spot where now her husband was kneeling in the street.

A neighbor intercepted her, hugged her, and would not let go. "Don't go over there," the woman told Pat. "Don't you go over there. Don't look."

27

Pat struggled briefly, then went limp. Then the tears came, in a sudden burst of anguish that was almost a wail. "That's my baby," she sobbed. "I've lost my baby."

"Don't you say that," the neighbor said. "You don't know that. We got to pray that he'll be all right." And right there, standing in the middle of Alabama Avenue, their arms around each other, the two women began to pray for the life of little David Myers.

◆ ◆ ◆

Thirty feet from the emergency entrance, tucked out of sight behind the emergency room main desk, is the Emergency Communications and Information Center, a name so bureaucratic and unpronounceable that everyone calls it the ECIC, or simply the radio room. It is a small room, made smaller by the enormous communications console that spans the length of one wall, and made cramped by the six-foot-high racks of electronic equipment lining the opposite wall. Two people can sit comfortably at the communications desk; anyone else has to stand, and usually has to move out of the way before long. It is a functional, no-nonsense place, as befits the nerve center of a regional trauma hospital.

Children's Hospital National Medical Center, being the only acute-care children's hospital in Washington, is the designated place to take injured children from the District and its suburbs. The statement is deceptive: To the casual observer it seems only natural that injured kids should go to a hospital for kids. If kids didn't require special treatment, why would we have pediatricians?

The reality is less clear and more political. It has, in many cases, been a fight to get other hospitals to admit that hurt children would do best at Children's Hospital. In an era of cost cutting and cutthroat competition among hospitals, no hospital willingly gives up a high-revenue patient, and hurt kids are high-revenue patients. So, no committees came calling on Children's Hospital to ask if they would please arrange to treat all the injured kids from around the nation's capital. No governmental body held hearings and concluded that hurt kids belonged at Children's Hospital. No army of parents marched and paraded to demand the best care for their kids. Children's Hospital became the designated pediatric trauma center because Marty Eichelberger understood the realities of the trauma business, and because Marty Eichelberger has two kids of his own.

To be taken seriously as a trauma center, you absolutely must start out with two things. One is a helipad; the other is a round-the-clock communications center. The ECIC was one of the first visible signs that Children's was getting into the trauma business, and it continues to be one of the mainstays of the operation, which is why, at three o'clock on a Sunday afternoon, Dave Hunter was hunched over the communications console, filling out forms.

Half an hour before, a helicopter had arrived bearing a young boy who'd nearly hung himself. Nobody had any idea whether it was an accident or a deliberate act; such cases always took days to sort out. In the trauma business, though, it is routine to assume the worst, so Dave was busy getting down all the details in writing. There would be lots of people, both inside and outside the hospital, who'd want to review his reports on this one. What a pain.

Dave chafed at being on the inside; in his home state of Minnesota, he was a fully trained and fully qualified cardiac rescue technician, the highest level a paramedic can reach. Then he'd moved to Maryland, and discovered that as far as the Maryland emergency medical system was concerned, the only way he'd be riding in the back of an ambulance was as a patient. All his training in Minnesota didn't count in Maryland; if he wanted to be certified in Maryland, he'd have to take all the courses all over again. No, he couldn't just take the test, that was against the rules. Modern-day emergency medicine was invented in Maryland, twenty-five years ago, and in the ensuing years the state's EMS system has become large and bureaucratic. Sorry, they told Dave Hunter; we don't have reciprocity with Minnesota.

So, instead of being out in the field providing care, Dave had joined the ECIC staff at Children's, where at least he could talk on the radio to the "field providers" while he made up his mind what to do about all the silly rules.

No fewer than seven different forms have to be filled out for every "trauma stat" admission at Children's. There is a standard trauma admission form, and a trauma log, and a traumatic injury severity scoring form, and a transport report. Dave hunched over his pile of papers. In front of him, muted sounds came from the various radio monitors. To the casual listener, the police and fire radio speakers emit a constant garble; only after many hours of listening does the garble become intelligible.

And only after many hundreds of hours of listening does the listening become so automatic that a person can do other things simultaneously, and even then it is difficult. Dave's head jerked when he heard the words "child struck" on the police radio, but he hadn't heard the location. He twisted dials on the console and listened intently. The paperwork could wait.

Finally, he picked up the signal of a District of Columbia Fire Department ambulance. The accident was at Twelfth Street and Alabama Avenue, in the southeast part of the city. Dave stuck his head out the door of the ECIC. "You might have another one," he said to Mary Hegenbarth, the pediatrician in charge of the emergency room on that particular Sunday. "Sounds like a pedestrian struck, in Southeast. I'll keep you posted."

Dave listened intently a while longer, twisting dials occasionally, but heard nothing. Finally he shrugged and went back to his paperwork. If anything were coming his way, they'd let him know. That, after all, was what a communications center was for.

◆ ◆ ◆

Someone in the crowd that formed around little David Myers put a hand on David Senior's shoulder. "Don't move him," the man said. "If his neck's broken, you'll hurt him if you move him." David Senior rocked back on his heels, then stood up, afraid, angry, frantic. He looked back at the Buick, still parked on the street. The front seat was empty now. That was good, he thought to himself; he wasn't sure he wanted to know who had hit his son. Then, just beyond the car, he spotted Pat, crying, being held by some woman.

The thought flashed through David's mind that not only had he just lost his son, he had probably lost his wife as well. What wife, after all, would have a man who turned his back on his son and let the boy get hit by a car? Then a second thought tumbled over the first: I've got to call her mother! Whenever David and Pat had disagreed, it had been Pat's mother who could always make sense of things, patch things up. Pat's mother would know what to do now. She always knew what to do, and Pat always listened to her. He turned back to the cluster of people, and said to no one in general, "Don't let anyone touch him. I've got to make a phone call."

He started running back toward the apartment, then realized he'd locked himself out. He detoured toward Pat. "Let me have your keys," he said. "I've got to let your mother know." Pat said nothing, but fished into her purse and handed over her keys. Their eyes met only briefly, and the question was in her eyes, but she didn't voice it. This was not the time or the place. Their reckoning would come later.

David ran into the house, dialed the number that he knew by heart. One ring, two rings, three rings—where is she? At the tenth ring, he hung up. She must still be at church, David thought. If there was time, he'd try again. If not, he'd call from the hospital.

When he ran back outside, he could hear the wail of an approaching ambulance. What took them so long? he wondered. It's been forever. He raced back to the street, knelt beside his son. Little David's eyes were closed now, his breath still coming in slow, shallow gasps. He was alive, but how badly was he hurt?

The paramedics trotted up with a gurney, and one of them knelt beside David. The boy's eyes were still closed; the medic lifted each eyelid once, then again. He lifted an arm, pressed a finger into little David's hand. "Anybody know the boy's name?" he asked.

"It's David," said David Senior. "I'm his father."

"David!" the paramedic said sharply. "David! Squeeze my hand! David! Listen to me, David! Squeeze my hand! David, your father's right here! Squeeze my hand, David!"

David Senior shifted around so he could get a better view. He was about to add his own exhortations to those of the paramedic when the medic let go of the boy's hand and fixed a stethoscope in his ears. He slid the disk inside the boy's shirt, listened for a long moment, then looked up. "I don't want to move him," he said to his partner. Then, to David's father, he added, "We don't have the equipment on board to immobilize him. If he's got a broken neck and we move him, we could paralyze him." Turning to his partner again, he said, "He needs to go to Children's. We need somebody to help package him, and we need the Park Police to transport him." The ambulance driver nodded, then did a slow, 360-degree turn, surveying the terrain for a place where a Park Police helicopter could land. Then he trotted off toward the ambulance.

A fire truck accompanied the second ambulance, putting the finishing touches on the Alabama Avenue traffic jam. Several District of Columbia police cars had also arrived, and two of them had parked across Alabama Avenue, while a third blocked off Twelfth Street. The crowd of spectators, which continued to grow in size, was now restricted to the two sidewalks while four ambulance medics and four firemen dashed back and forth between the second ambulance and the spot where little David lay, an oxygen mask covering his face, still unconscious, still not moving.

As soon as the second ambulance arrived, the new paramedic went through the same "Squeeze my finger!" routine as the first. But then, when he grabbed a hunk of David's forearm between his fingers and pinched, little David jerked the arm back. "That's a good sign," he said.

Another medic brought over three pink plastic neck collars, each a different size. The senior medic selected one, then grasped little David's chin on both sides and carefully, gently, hauled back on the little head while his partner fitted the collar around the neck, then strapped it into place. "Okay, now the backboard," the medic said. The backboard, a flat, coffin-shaped piece of heavy plywood with straps attached to it, was already on the street beside little David. Three sets of hands gently rolled David off the pavement and onto the backboard.

"Gimme a minute now," the medic instructed, fitting a stethoscope to his ears. A blood-pressure cuff had already been wrapped around one of David's arms, and now the medic reinflated it, listening intently to David's lower arm with his stethoscope. "I think we ought to put him in MAST trousers," the medic said. One of the firemen trotted off toward the ambulance.

Military anti-shock trousers are one of the current controversies in trauma medicine everywhere, and pediatric trauma medicine in particular. "Trauma pants" are fashioned after the G-suits worn by pilots. The bulky trousers have inflatable panels along the legs and abdomen; when pumped up, they squeeze hard on the lower extremities, forcing more blood up into the torso. For a pilot, this means more blood available to pump to the brain, lessening the chance of a blackout. For a trauma patient, it means more blood available to the body's critical organs, including the brain. If a patient has serious internal bleeding, MAST trousers can buy him a few more minutes, critical minutes in the race to the hospital.

There is an additional benefit: MAST trousers are very effective for splinting broken legs, and for holding back the bleeding that can accompany a fracture of the upper leg. Many trauma scientists have studied the use of MAST trousers, and some have come to the conclusion that they make no difference in the patient's ultimate outcome.

But ambulance men—the field providers—find them useful, and in trauma medicine the opinions of the field providers outweigh the opinions of the theoreticians.

It took several minutes to assemble the trauma pants, maneuvering the pieces into place, then zipping them along little David's legs, testing David's blood pressure, inflating the trauma pants a panel at a time, testing the blood pressure each time. It was partly deliberate and partly killing time waiting for the helicopter. Parents and crowds, the medics knew, like to see you doing something.

As they finished inflating the last panel, the sound of the chopper appeared distantly, then grew rapidly in volume. The medics quickly wrapped a blanket around little David, buckled him onto the backboard with the nylon web straps, and stood to watch as the helicopter made a rapid circle over the area at an altitude no more than one hundred feet, then settled to a landing on a small patch of grass on the grounds of St. Elizabeth's Psychiatric Hospital.

A tall man wearing blue coveralls and a pistol in a shoulder holster ran to the wrought-iron fence separating St. Elizabeth's from Alabama Avenue. The senior ambulance medic met him, and the two men conferred a moment. Then the medic ran back to the scene. "We can't hand him over the fence, and they can't land here," the medic said. "Let's get him in the ambulance and drive him around."

David's parents had stood quietly, arms around each other, watching. The police had allowed them closer than the rest of the crowd, but had kept them from coming too close. Now one of the ambulance men approached them. "We have to drive him around," he said, pointing at the helicopter. "As soon as we get him to the helicopter, we'll take both of you to the hospital to be with him."

"Can you tell how bad he's hurt?" asked David Senior.

"I'm not a doctor," the medic answered, "but I can tell it's serious. That's why we want to get him to Children's Hospital. If anybody can help him, they can."

The ambulance men worked rapidly but carefully. With the police clearing the way, they backed an ambulance close to where little David lay; then they gently lifted the gurney to waist height, rolled it across the short stretch of pavement to the back of the ambulance, slid it in, and locked it into place. The ambulance cruised off down the street to the St. Elizabeth's gate a block away. Then it doubled back, on the other side of the fence, and stopped twenty feet from the whirring blades of the helicopter. The men jumped out, unloaded the gurney and, heads bent low, pulled the gurney up alongside the chopper. The helicopter medic helped the ambulance men guide little David, backboard and all, into place on the chopper's port side. The ambulance men retreated, the medic ran around to the other side of the helicopter and got in, and the noise of the blades suddenly increased from a loud drone to a piercing whine. The whine became thunder, and the chopper lifted, slowly first, then rapidly into the sky and, like a great clattering metallic angel of mercy, vanished over the rooftops.

"Sit here," the ambulance medic said to David's parents, pointing at two narrow benches in the back of the ambulance. "As soon as we get packed up, we'll take you to Children's."

◆ ◆ ◆

Dave Hunter had long since finished his paperwork and was now reading a book. He'd listened off and on for a good half hour without hearing any indication that anything had come of the Alabama Avenue pedestrian accident. Finally, he'd decided that either his ears were deceiving him or, as sometimes happened, that it was either a false alarm, or the child had been killed outright. Either way, that first call was now almost an hour old, and you can't stay at red alert all the time. He'd almost forgotten even hearing the call when the speaker on his radio console suddenly came to life: "Eagle One to Children's."

Dave swung his chair upright. I bet this is it, he thought. "This is Children's, Eagle One."

"Eagle One. Children's, we're en route with a four-year-old pedestrian, serious head injury, unconscious, and posturing, ETA two minutes."

"Okay, Eagle One, we'll be waiting." As he spoke, he grabbed for the telephone. In the same instant that he released the radio microphone button, he spoke into the phone. "Trauma stat. Helipad. One minute."

At the other end of the telephone, the hospital page operator pressed a large red button on her paging console and simultaneously, all over the hospital, nineteen red beepers came alive with the special "trauma stat" alert tone, a blend of bosun's whistle and jet airplane. Nurses, residents, lab technicians, and X-ray technicians stopped what they were doing and headed for the first floor. *Stat* is a word medical people use. It means now. This instant. Immediately. Many of the trauma team members were hurrying down hallways and toward stairways even before the page operator repeated Dave's words: "Trauma stat. Helipad. One minute. Trauma stat. Helipad. One minute."

◆ ◆ ◆

Even without the markings, you can spot the Park Police helicopters by the way they fly them: fast and hard. The Children's Hospital helipad is close to the building, and Maryland State Police pilots like to settle in gradually, testing for any possible updrafts that might make for a rough landing. The Park Police fly their craft straight in, circling and descending at the same time, so that at the end of the approach sweep, the chopper is on the helipad, with no time wasted in hovering. The maneuver, besides showing off the pilot's skill with his craft, emphasizes the urgent nature of the flight.

By the time Eagle One landed, a resident, a nurse, an ER technician, and a security guard were standing alongside the helipad, an empty gurney waiting to receive the patient. As soon as the chopper touched the ground, the pilot unpitched his rotor blades, flattening them so they no longer bit into the air. This changed the sound of the bird, and that change in sound was the trauma team's cue to dash forward, heads down, pulling the gurney toward the side of the helicopter.

The helicopter medic walked around the nose of the bird and helped open the special doors to expose the stretcher inside. The medic undid the heavy web straps that held the passenger in place, and then five sets of hands lifted the patient, still strapped to the backboard, out of the helicopter and on to the gurney. Immediately, the nurse applied a clear, green plastic mask to the patient's face. As the doctor and the ER technician began to pull the gurney across the helipad, the nurse trotted behind the stretcher, holding the oxygen mask in place. The helicopter medic walked to the pilot's window, shouted something over the noise of the blades, then turned to follow the trauma team, trotting to catch up.

Five _____

In the jargon of the Children's Hospital staff, *code* originally was a short form of *code blue,* which is an emergency alert that a child has stopped breathing. With use, the noun turned into a verb, and then there were stories of kids who "coded" up on 3-Green. Soon *code* came to be a generic term for every sort of life-threatening crisis; it was only natural, then, that the special room in the emergency suite reserved for critically hurt trauma cases began to be called the code room. The name has stuck.

Dr. Eichelberger's province has grown in recent years, and now there are two code rooms. Code Room Number Two is closer to the helipad by perhaps ten feet, but that tiny time advantage makes it the code room of preference.

The gurney bearing little David Myers slid into place in the code room, guided by the helipad team. A respiratory technician pressed a black rubber mask hard against the boy's face, feeding pure oxygen to his lungs. The anesthesiologist, standing beside the respiratory technician, glanced at the wall clock and jotted down the time: 2:55 P.M.

Many things began to happen simultaneously. Trauma medicine is, above all, checklist medicine. When a child has been hit by a car, you assume the worst. Assume everything on your checklist, and one by one, rule it out or treat it. A quiet panic settled over the trauma team as each member began to work down his list.

Standing near the foot of the bed, Mary Fallat, M.D., worked down her own mental checklist. As chief surgical resident at Children's Hospital, she is designated as the "surgical coordinator" in trauma cases. She has no specific medical chore to perform; it is her job to coordinate the efforts of all the others. When no chief surgical resident is available, the attending physician from the ER is in charge. When Mary Fallat is in the room, she is the boss.

She listened intently as the helicopter medic recited what he knew of David's recent medical history: "This is David; he's a four-year-old male pedestrian struck by an automobile and thrown fifty feet. He has been unconscious and unresponsive since the accident. On arrival of the first ambulance his pupils were fixed and unequal, left greater than right. He's been breathing on his own the whole time, but it's very abnormal breathing, although his breath sounds are clear. His blood pressure has been stable. He has bilateral closed femur fractures inside the MAST trousers. He has no known medical history and no known allergies. His parents were at the scene and are on their way here now."

Fallat smiled and nodded to the medic. These guys were good. The history had been brief and concise, with no editorializing, no waffling. If only she could teach her residents to do that, morning rounds would be over in half the time. With that history, they had a good head start on figuring out what was wrong with little David.

Her first concern as coordinator was for David's head. The trauma team could take care of the rest. She peered around the door of the code room, caught the eye of the assistant director of nursing, standing just outside. "Neuro?" she said.

"On the way," the nurse replied.

"Thanks." Fallat stepped back inside, moved to the foot of the bed, and watched the trauma team perform.

On the right side of the bed, a surgical resident listened intently with a stethoscope to both sides of David's chest, moving the disk of the stethoscope several times. He looked at the anesthesiologist and respiratory technician at the head of the bed. "Breath sounds are okay," he reported. That part was good; the jerky, unrhythmic breathing was not. Something was wrong, and they'd have to figure it out, but for the moment they knew from the breath sounds that the airway was clear. If the boy's lungs were collapsing, or filling with his own blood, the breath sounds wouldn't be there at all. Airway, breathing, and circulation, one, two, three, in that order. Airway and breathing were okay for the moment. Now for circulation. The resident quickly swabbed the inside of David's arm with foaming brown antiseptic, located a large vein, and threaded an IV needle into it. The nurse at his side took over, taping the needle firmly into place and attaching it to a bag of clear fluid, which she then hung on a rack above the bed. The surgical resident, meanwhile, began helping nurse-right place EKG leads on the boy's chest.

On the left side of the bed, a resident from the ICU paused while the nurse at his side pumped up a blood-pressure cuff on David's upper arm. Then he quickly and expertly drew a blood sample. He filled five small vials with blood; as each one was filled, he held it out, without looking, and another nurse took it from him and labeled it. When the fifth vial was full, the nurse put all five vials in a plastic bag, walked to the code room doorway, and handed the blood samples to a waiting lab technician. The lab tech moved off down the hallway at a brisk trot. Meanwhile, the ICU resident carefully removed the needle from David's arm, pressed a gauze pad on the spot for a long moment to stop the bleeding, then moved back. The nurse with the blood-pressure cuff moved in with her stethoscope, listened intently for a moment. "One fourteen over sixty-one," she announced. The clock on the wall read 2:57. Two minutes postadmission, little David's vital signs were stable.

There was no guarantee they would stay that way, though. That was one of the disadvantages of MAST trousers. They could mask a serious injury and artificially stabilize a patient by forcing blood up into the torso, and then when you deflated the trousers and the blood rushed back into the legs, blooie! You had a mess on your hands. Standing at the foot of the bed, Mary Fallat spoke to the left-side resident: "Go ahead and start your IV before we take down the MAST trousers." With two IV lines in place, they'd be better able to compensate, if David's blood pressure began to drop suddenly.

Fallat reached out and touched David's left foot. It looked gray and felt cold to the touch. Not good. That could be the MAST trousers, or it could be that the sharp edges of the broken femur had torn the large artery that serves the leg. If the latter were true, then David would have a rough time when the trauma pants came off. The pressure would be holding back the bleeding, but as soon as they deflated the trousers, there'd be exciting times in the code room.

Minutes are precious in the code room, but Fallat decided this was a good time to stall, at least until the neurosurgeon arrived. If David started to go sour on them, they'd have to give him all manner of drugs, all of which would interfere with neuro's ability to judge how badly his brain had been hurt. It couldn't be that much longer now.

◆ ◆ ◆

Outside the code room, out of the way but instantly available, the other members of the trauma team waited their turns. An X-ray technician lounged against the wall alongside her huge lumbering portable X-ray machine. A lab technician sat on a desk in one of the offices, waiting for more blood samples. A security guard moved around, trying to look busy. The clerk from the front desk in the emergency room, her job long since completed, hung around anyway, peering into the code room from time to time. The regular *peep-peep-peep* of the heart monitor could be heard all through the hallway.

When the man in the immaculate white lab coat approached, the crew took note, but no one jumped to attention. Even on a Sunday afternoon, it wasn't that unusual for Dr. Eichelberger to show up during a trauma admission. He greeted each member of the team, shook hands with the lab technician, and nodded to the neurosurgery resident who breezed past him on his way into the code room. Dr. Eichelberger did not enter the code room; rules are rules. Sauntering over to the nursing director, just outside the door to the code room, he asked, quietly, "Whatcha got?"

"Head injury," the nurse replied. "Bad one, it looks like."

"Parents here?"

"On the way. So is social work. We notified them."

"Social work's not here?" Eichelberger asked. The nurse shook her head. "Great," he said bitterly. It was an old battle. Social work, perennially understaffed, couldn't keep people in the hospital on weekends; they had to settle for having social workers on call. Marty had tried again and again to have social work coverage extended to the weekends, but to no avail. When money is tight, the departments not directly involved in giving medical care—like social work—are the first to suffer.

That was a shortsighted view, in Eichelberger's opinion. It might be okay in an adult hospital, but children were different. When you have an injured child, you have an injured family, and you have to treat the whole family.

On weekdays, that mechanism is the social worker. When a hurt child comes in the door, he is met by the trauma team. When the family comes in, they are met by a social worker who answers their questions, provides them with a telephone, or a cup of coffee, or simply finds them a quiet, private place to cry. Most important, the social worker keeps the parents someplace distant, where they are spared the torment of listening to their child's screams.

The most worrisome thing about little David was that he wasn't making a sound. When the left-side resident drew the arterial blood sample, a procedure that hurts like hell, David's eyes fluttered, but he made no sound. That was a serious sign; drawing arterial blood can rouse even a semicomatose child. In the corner of the code room, the charge nurse made a note on her chart: "unresponsive to painful stimuli."

In the hallway outside, the emergency room desk clerk, who had slipped away when Dr. Eichelberger arrived, returned. "The parents are here," she announced quietly.

"Still no social work?" Eichelberger asked. The clerk shook her head. "Okay, I'll see if I can track one down."

♦ ♦ ♦

The neurosurgery resident shone lights in David's eyes, screamed in his ear, lifted both arms, pinched him, scraped his bare feet with the tip of his rubber hammer, and screamed in his ear again, all to no avail. The best response he could get was slight movement in response to pain. Whipping out his ophthalmoscope, he peeled back David's eyelids, one at a time, and peered into them, examining the backs of the eyeballs, where the optic nerve is attached to the retina. Both eyes were bloody. That was a bad sign. An impact strong enough to tear the retinas was also strong enough to bounce the brain around inside the skull, bruising it and causing it to swell. Inside a closed skull, the brain can only swell a little before it begins to choke off its own blood supply or worse, before it starts to squeeze itself downward, out the small opening where the spine is attached.

"Give him about seven and a half of mannitol," the neuro man announced, "and let's do a CT of the head."

"Do you mind if we intubate him now?" Fallat asked. "I really don't like his breathing at all."

"Is the C-spine clear?" asked the neurosurgeon. Examining the neck for possible spine fractures was a semisacred part of the trauma routine. There is little to be gained in saving a child's life if, in the process, you mishandle a neck injury and make the child a quadriplegic. At the moment, little David's neck was held rigid by a plastic collar. If he had a broken neck, the collar would keep his spine straight and a little stretched, the ideal position for preventing any additional damage to the spinal cord.

But the cervical collar made it difficult to put a tube down David's windpipe. And David wasn't breathing well on his own. One of the ways you treat brain swelling is to put the patient on a respirator and give him lots of pure oxygen. And in this case, the neurosurgeon was more worried about David's brain than his neck. However . . .

"Let me hold his head while you intubate him," the neurosurgeon said, walking around to the head of the bed. As the surgical resident began unstrapping the neck collar, the neurosurgeon grabbed both sides of David's head and began to apply steady, even pressure, keeping the neck stretched and straight.

"Two of Surital and two of Atropine, please," the anesthesiologist announced. Surital is an anesthetic, and atropine causes a rapid heartbeat. Both are part of the standard armamentarium of the anesthesiologist. Together, they make it easier to thread the large-bore plastic tube down into the trachea. The medications nurse rapidly drew two syringes and injected the drugs directly into the IV line in David's left arm. After a few moments' wait, David became noticeably more limp.

A laryngoscope is like a large curved metal tongue depressor with a handle on one end, and a flashlight built into the handle. There isn't a sharp edge or even a corner anywhere on the business end of the device; it is designed to slide into the patient's mouth, lift the collapsed tongue up off the back of the throat, and, lighting its own way down back of the throat, part the limp vocal cords so that the breathing tube can be maneuvered past them without damage.

It was clumsy work; the anesthesiologist had to reach around the neurosurgeon, and it took three tries before he finally got the laryngoscope properly aligned. Then he rapidly threaded the air pipe into place, withdrew the laryngoscope, and relaxed. "One hundred of succs, please." "Succs" is short for *succinylcholine,* a paralyzing drug like curare. Nobody ever pronounces the entire word. With the endotracheal tube in place, the anesthesiologist could take over David's breathing for him. Now it was safe to paralyze him, which was the best possible way to guarantee that some random muscle spasm wouldn't cause him to move his neck. David wasn't moving anyway, but just to be sure, the neurosurgeon held his grip on the sides of

David's head until well after the medications nurse had injected the succs into David's intravenous line. Then he replaced the plastic collar.

Mary Fallat took a deep breath. "Okay," she announced. "As soon as we get him out of the MAST trousers, we can take him upstairs."

◆ ◆ ◆

Mirean Coleman isn't there on weekends, but her office gets used as the parents' waiting room. Mr. and Mrs. Myers sat, alone, on the orange couch. David Senior sat hunched over, staring at the floor. Patricia stared straight ahead. Finally, without moving her eyes, Patricia asked the inevitable question.

"What happened?"

David's voice was quiet, defeated. "I thought you were right behind me. When I heard the door, I thought it was you coming in, not him going out."

David paused. Pat said nothing. Finally David spoke again. "I was upstairs. I had turned on the television. David said, 'Where Mommy?' and I said, 'Mommy's downstairs.' And he ran down the stairs. . . ." His voice broke. Pat looked directly at him for the first time; his eyes brimmed with tears. "And when I came out the door, I could see him lying in the street." He shook his head; tears splashed on the floor.

Pat looked at him. His hands were clasped tightly in front of him. She reached over, unthreaded the tensed fingers, and took one hand tightly in hers. "We have to pray," she said.

◆ ◆ ◆

The scary part about deflating MAST trousers is right at the beginning. If you are going to have a problem, it is going to be as soon as you start reducing the pressure on the trousers. Mary Fallat glanced up again to make sure both IV lines were in place and working before she finally undid the valve on the left trouser leg, released the pressure slightly, then closed the valve again. She grasped David's left foot, feeling for a pulse. This time, the pulse was stronger. That was good; that probably meant that the big femoral artery in the upper leg was okay. But no guarantees.

One of the devices in Code Room Number Two is an automatic blood-pressure machine. Once you put the cuff and sensors on the patient's arm, you can set the machine to take pulse and blood pressure at any interval. Now Mary directed the nurse who tended the machine to set it to thirty-second intervals. If David's blood pressure began to drop significantly, they'd have to begin giving him lots of extra fluid, which wouldn't be good for his swelling brain but would at least keep him alive until they could get him to surgery.

The blood-pressure reading dropped from 116 to 107 in the first thirty-second interval. Everyone in the code room stood quietly and watched the blood-pressure monitor. The third reading was 107. So was the fourth. People began to breathe again. A small drop in blood pressure meant a relatively small amount of bleeding in David's upper legs. Certainly, if the femoral artery had been severed, they'd have known it by now. Score one for little David.

The assistant director of nursing came to the doorway of the code room. "H and H eleven point six and thirty-five point seven," she announced. The two numbers told the team that David's supply of red blood cells, while adequate, was slightly below normal. This, too, was consistent with relatively minor bleeding. Mary Fallat opened the valve on the MAST trousers again, deflated them by two-thirds. Then another pause to watch the blood-pressure machine. The blood pressure dropped to 105, then to 102, then went back to 106, then 118. Fallat let the remaining pressure out of the MAST trousers, and began to unfasten them. The medical resident drew another blood sample. As soon as the MAST trousers were off, Fallat called to the nursing director, "Ready for X-ray."

The code room checklist was far from complete, but now that Mary Fallat was convinced that David was stable, she quietly slipped out of the code room. As the highest-ranking physician, she had another responsibility: talking to the parents.

Fallat stopped at the emergency room desk, where the clerk pointed her to the room where David's parents were waiting. She paused a moment outside the door to gather her thoughts, then went in.

David and Patricia Myers sat, together, on the orange plastic couch. "Mr. and Mrs. Myers?" Fallat asked. They nodded. "I'm Dr. Fallat." Mr. and Mrs. Myers nodded, mumbled greetings, and waited.

Nowhere in medical school, nowhere during residency, indeed, nowhere in medicine are there formal instructions on how a physician should deal with the patient's family. It is something a physician learns (or fails to learn) from his fellow physicians; each has his own approach, and each is unique. Mary Fallat is formal but gentle, compassionate but matter-of-fact.

"Your son," she began without preamble, "has been hurt very badly. He is unconscious, and there is probably some injury to his brain. We don't know how much, yet. In a little while, we're going to take him upstairs for a CAT scan; that should tell us more.

"He had trouble breathing, so we've put a tube in his windpipe and we're breathing for him. Our initial X-rays suggest that his lungs were bruised in the accident; if that's true, he'll need to be on a respirator for several days."

Mr. Myers broke in. "Will he—" he caught himself. "How long will his recovery period be?"

Dr. Fallat hesitated an instant, deciding which question to answer. "Assuming everything else goes well, his leg injuries would keep him here the longest," she said. "Both his legs are broken; the right one is broken about here," she pointed on her own leg, "and will be more of a problem because the fracture is so near the hip. The left one is closer to the knee, and will be easier to manage. I would say that ordinarily with two broken femurs you should expect a hospital stay of four to six weeks, maybe even a little longer."

Mr. and Mrs. Myers looked at each other but remained silent.

"I can tell you some good things: His blood pressure has remained stable so far, and that's a good sign. We got the X-rays on his neck, and it's fine. There's apparently no extensive bleeding in his legs. He had the inflatable trousers on his legs just in case; we took them off and everything seems okay. The next thing now is to move him up to CAT scan and see if we can learn more about his head injury."

She glanced from one to the other. "That's what we know so far. Do either of you have any questions?"

Mrs. Myers opened her mouth to speak, but her husband spoke first. "What are his chances of surviving?" The question was flat, uninflected, bleak.

"I can answer that question a lot better after we've done the CAT scans," Dr. Fallat said carefully. "He does have a very bad head injury; just how bad we don't know yet. I would say that the next twenty-four hours are critical; we'll be in a lot better position to predict the outcome after that time." She hadn't exactly evaded the question, but she hadn't exactly answered it either. The truth was that right then nobody, not even Mary Fallat, had any idea whether little David would live or die.

Six

It is impossible to talk of trauma without also talking of politics, and of money.

Years ago, when there were no trauma centers, hospitals competed for accident victims on a more or less even footing. Attracting patients was a fairly straightforward matter of bribing the ambulance drivers. It was not done overtly, of course; the bribes took the form of free food, or free supplies, or perhaps direct financial support for the ambulance service. Sometimes all a hospital needed to do was assign its prettiest nurses to the emergency room. The competition for patients was there, but it was quiet, genteel, and noticeable only by insiders.

The competition made some doctors uneasy. Medicine, they had been taught, was more than a business; it was a profession, a brotherhood founded on mutual respect and unity of purpose. If the community of healers were subjected to the pressures of the marketplace, the community of man would suffer.

But compete they did. Accident victims were the most attractive of patients. True, the trauma cases usually arrived at odd hours, and sometimes they wrecked the entire hospital's routine for a day, but on the other hand, trauma patients were usually lucrative. An accident victim required laboratory tests, X-rays, EKGs, consultations by specialists, surgery, blood, respiratory therapy, intensive care, painkillers, antibiotics, and physical therapy. Virtually everyone in the hospital had a piece of the case. Best of all, trauma victims usually had insurance. Even when they died, someone paid their bills.

The brotherhood of physicians preferred to leave such grubby details to administrators, but the economics were undeniable: Trauma patients were very desirable patients.

Then a few bold surgeons began to suggest that accident victims would fare better if they were taken to large hospitals that had all the necessary manpower, equipment, and supplies close at hand. The surgeons produced statistics to prove that accident victims survived more often at large hospitals than at small ones. Then they proposed that the largest hospitals begin treating all the trauma cases. When the brotherhood of healers resisted this idea, the surgeons sidestepped them and went directly to the politicians, who viewed the saving of lives as a worthwhile goal. Thus the first regional trauma centers were born.

And thus began the rift, subtle but real, within the brotherhood of healers. On one side are the trauma doctors, men whose desire to save lives led them again and again to violate their profession's unwritten old-boy code of conduct. On the other side are the old boys, perturbed by these brash young surgeons who made up their own rules and ignored the advice of their betters.

The years have vindicated the traumatologists, of course; the statistical proof has become overwhelming: Trauma victims survive better at trauma centers. Trauma is a surgical disease. Its victims usually bleed to death; for them, time is critical. They must be treated by bold men with knives, not thoughtful men with stethoscopes. The men with stethoscopes acknowledge this now, but only grudgingly.

Once the politicians got involved, they stayed involved. Committees were appointed, meetings held, plans drawn. Ambulance attendants became paramedics, with hundreds of hours of specialized training in what came to be called "prehospital care." State agencies were given the authority to certify hospitals as qualified trauma centers, and ambulance services rewrote their rules to stipulate that anyone who appeared to be seriously hurt should go to a trauma center.

The competition between hospitals began to emerge into plain sight. Hospitals added trauma bays to their emergency rooms, hired trauma surgeons, and applied to the state agencies for certification to treat those wonderful patients for whom somebody's insurance always paid. Trauma became a growth industry.

And inside hospitals, the polite, scholarly, cutthroat rivalry continued. Medicare and Medicaid imposed strict limits on how long a patient could stay in the hospital. Blue Cross began tightening the screws on inpatient treatment costs. Occupancy began to fall; hospitals everywhere had empty beds. Budget priority began to follow the docs who could fill beds with paying patients.

The trauma surgeons notified their friends, the politicians, that if length-of-stay restrictions were applied to trauma patients, nobody would want to treat them and some of them would die. The politicians obligingly exempted trauma from cost-containment regulations.

Trauma surgeons began to gain the attention of hospital executives, along with the renewed ill will of their colleagues, who could only watch, seething, as the traumatologists sliced off a bit of this department, a chunk of that one, and half of someone else's, incorporating ever more beds, floor space, and budget money into their little trauma fiefdoms, all in the name of saving lives. Saving lives! It was an absolute, invincible cloak in which to drape the lust for empire. The statistics were unarguable. The politics were unarguable. The morality was unarguable. But the bottom line was money; the trauma surgeons were getting it all, and their colleagues resented it. They still do.

There are still physicians at Children's Hospital National Medical Center who resent Marty Eichelberger as an upstart, an interloper, and an empire builder. Learned colleagues, men far senior to Dr. Eichelberger, have opposed the expansion of the trauma service into a hospitalwide interdisciplinary program headed, of course, by Dr. Eichelberger.

Part of this may be a function of the Marty Eichelberger personality. Like many surgeons, Marty has the air of a man always in a hurry. His staff jokes that he spends most of his life "in warp drive." When you see him, he is nearly always on his way to or from someplace, and in a hurry. Members of his own staff gripe periodically about their lack of access and have been known simply to corner the man in a hallway and physically prevent him from moving until some particular problem has been discussed and resolved.

Some of his resentful colleagues would do well to employ the same tactics. When cornered, Marty is not above compromise, and since he began building his trauma service in 1980, he has repeatedly compromised on what he considers minor matters of protocol and ego, usually as a means to bringing an end to some subterranean turf war. He will compromise on anything, he says—anything except matters affecting patient care.

Many of the earliest controversies, quite naturally, involved his approach to patient care. One of the few tactics available to a resentful brotherhood is to complain that trauma protocols are overaggressive, or worse, ineffective. So, since 1981, Marty Eichelberger has systematically gathered large amounts of statistical information on every young accident victim who comes through the door, and his numbers have consistently borne out every one of his edicts on patient care.

But while Marty's numbers and his forceful ways may not have won him any popularity contests among the physicians into whose specialties he has intruded with his trauma service, the program has won considerable favor with the hospital's board of directors and its administrators, because the statistics also clearly show that Dr. Eichelberger is a rainmaker, a revenue provider, and getting better at it all the time.

When he first came to Children's Hospital in 1980, the emergency room's clientele consisted largely of acutely ill children from the poor neighborhoods of Washington. This, to borrow an administrator's phrase, did not constitute a "good payor mix." The patients were nearly all insured by Medicaid, the government program that provides medical assistance to poor people. Medicaid pays slowly and reluctantly, and it never pays the entire bill. The emergency room stayed busy all the time, but it was not a money-maker for the hospital.

Marty had helped set up a trauma service at Philadelphia Children's Hospital, so he knew that the first step is simply to make the public, and especially the paramedics, aware that Children's was set up to handle seriously injured kids. Then, in the normal course of business, injured kids would begin to be brought there.

First, though, he needed a couple of trauma bays in the emergency room. To call yourself a trauma center, you have to have trauma bays, rooms reserved exclusively for the admission and resuscitation of trauma victims. The rooms have to be available twenty-four hours a day, and they have to be equipped with every conceivable piece of equipment that might be needed to handle every conceivable type of injury that may roll in the door.

That sort of setup is not free, and hospitals do not readily commit floor space, instruments, machines, and manpower without extremely good cause. Early in his tenure at Children's, Marty sat down with his boss, the chief of surgery, Dr. Judson G. Randolph. How, he asked, could they force the hospital to commit the resources necessary to maintain two trauma bays in the emergency room?

Dr. Randolph eyed this bright young surgeon who had come to him so highly recommended by Dr. Koop. Bright, yes; aggressive, yes; but there were, Dr. Randolph reflected, still things that the old bull could teach the young bull about pace. Dr. Randolph had fought similar battles twenty years before, when he arrived at Children's as its very first full-time pediatric surgeon. Today, pediatric surgery is a known and accepted specialty, but when Dr. Randolph was brand-new, so was the specialty, and he was shocked to discover that the established general surgeons around town, and especially the ones who practiced part-time at Children's Hospital, resented the implication that you couldn't be a good pediatric surgeon without special training. He was even more shocked the first time someone called him a communist because he worked for the hospital instead of being in private practice.

He overcame those obstacles sometimes by confronting them, sometimes by ignoring them, and sometimes by simply stepping around them. Today, Dr. Randolph is one of the premier figures in pediatric surgery, a charter member of many of its most distinguished societies, and author and editor of many of its most respected academic writings. But it didn't come free, and it wasn't always fun.

Neither had the building of a burn center for children been free, but Dr. Randolph had done it by forging alliances and overcoming the suspicion, mistrust, and outright opposition of other departments to put together a burn unit that was a model of multidisciplinary medical care. In the burn unit, the surgeons attended to the treatment of the burns, the pediatricians looked after the infections, physical therapists made sure injured limbs were exercised so they wouldn't tighten up and become useless, primary nurses planned the patient's daily treatment schedule, and dieticians planned high-calorie menus to provide the nutrients needed by a recovering burn patient. The system worked well, everyone agreed. It would be a good model for the trauma service.

"Why," asked Dr. Randolph, "don't we wait a while, and fight that battle when we have more ammunition?" He jotted a name on a slip of paper, handed it to Marty. The name was DeVore Trust.

"These people have been very helpful to us in the past," Dr. Randolph told Marty. "Why don't you put together a presentation for them, and a cost estimate, and we'll see if we can get them to help fund this program."

As it worked out, the DeVore Trust did something they'd never done before: They committed money for a teaching program to train paramedics in the field care of injured children. That, in turn, had a snowball effect within the Children's Hospital administration, and soon Dr. Eichelberger found himself with a budget for trauma research and development.

One of the first things Marty did was to hire Tom McGinley as a coordinator for acute trauma care. It was a natural choice; Eichelberger was a former Navy doctor, McGinley, a former Navy medic. They spoke the same language, agreed on the same goals.

And McGinley, like Eichelberger, was appalled by what he saw in the emergency room.

The place was oriented to treating medical emergencies like colds and flu, asthma, dehydration resulting from diarrhea, poison ivy, minor burns, ingestion of things that required stomach pumping, and the like. Despite the crowding that often produced a bus-station environment in the ER waiting room, the place functioned well at those things, which meant it functioned well 98 percent of the time.

When a serious trauma case came in, though, it was a different story.

One classic management lecture talks about the difference between a ballet and a rugby match. In a ballet, everyone knows exactly where to stand and what moves to make. Every time you dance the ballet you do it the same way. Everybody works from the same script; all the kinks have been worked out in advance, during rehearsals, and everybody knows how it will come out.

In a rugby match you have rules, but nothing is rehearsed, so each game is made up as it goes along. By the time it is over, there are always a couple of people hurt, a couple of people angry, a couple of people thrown out for penalties, and so on.

To McGinley's eye, the emergency room's response to trauma fit the rugby match analogy perfectly. In a moderately serious case, the pediatricians who ran the emergency room would call for a surgical consultation. There are surgical residents in the hospital twenty-four hours a day, so finding a surgeon was usually not a problem. But when the surgeon got to the emergency room, he often had to send runners for the clamps, sutures, special needles, or whatever else he needed to treat a particular injury.

In the really severe cases, it was possible to muster a great deal of medical talent in a short time by sounding a code blue from the emergency room. This would bring, depending on the time of day, somewhere between fifteen and twenty-five people to the emergency room, every one of them at a dead run. The resulting scene, as two dozen people converged on the treatment room and all tried to help at the same time, was more suggestive of a rugby scrum than a learned consultation among medical colleagues.

The first thing McGinley did was write voluminous descriptions of the problems he saw, along with suggestions for improving the situation. Then, one by one, he and Marty set out to implement the suggestions.

The very first thing they did was help the emergency room staff set up two trauma bays and stock them with all the proper tools and supplies necessary to treat serious trauma. They were, of course, surgical tools and supplies. That done, Eichelberger and McGinley faded into the background to watch the results.

The results were impressive. Emergencies requiring the attention of a surgeon began to progress more smoothly. Had they been gathering the numbers at the time, they would have seen a statistical improvement: shorter stays in the ER, shorter stays in the hospital. The first law of trauma is that the quicker you can fix what's wrong with a trauma patient, the sooner he will be well enough to go home. The unofficial trauma service had racked up one invisible victory.

McGinley and Eichelberger jokingly referred to the trauma service as a "submarine service." It had no legal existence; no "trauma service" was listed on any hospital organizational chart. Yet from time to time it would surface; Tom McGinley would come sauntering through the emergency room and announce that he was from the trauma service and was there to help.

The emergency room staff had to admit it *did* help. When McGinley and Eichelberger proposed that they follow a checklist and gave them a sample, they tried it and it worked. When he suggested that a trauma team, separate from a code blue team, be designated and given its own special call-down code, that, too, made sense. And given the checklist and the team, it only made sense to organize the team so that the items on the checklist—they called it a "treatment protocol"—were divided up evenly among team members. That way everyone had a role, and the checklist got completed a lot faster. The people who didn't have to be inside the code room—the X-ray technician, the lab technicians, the blood bank technicians, the social worker—all were designated as the "outer core," or support group. They would stand outside the code room door, out of the way but instantly available when needed. The inner core consisted of just those nurses and residents necessary to work through the checklist. It was a highly practical setup, with the surgical resident on the patient's right side, the medical resident on the patient's left, and the anesthesiologist at the head of the bed—remarkably like the inside of an operating room. The surgical resident, of course, would be in charge.

The other absolute of building a trauma service is building a database. Twenty-five years ago in Baltimore, R. Adams Cowley steamrollered his opponents with numbers that proved his way was better. If the trauma service at Children's Hospital was ever going to change from submarine to fortress, it would be done with numbers.

So it was that Dr. Elmer Antonio Mangubat, who came to Children's to do a brief trauma research stint during a break in his surgical residency, stayed on as a permanent "research fellow" for the next five years.

Tony Mangubat had an uncanny grasp of numbers and an equally impressive knowledge of computers. Somehow, Marty scrounged up the money to purchase a pair of IBM PCs, and Marty Eichelberger's database came to life. Mangubat had become bored with his surgical residency long before he came to Children's; he was anxious for a chance to do something new, perhaps work on a Ph.D. to go with his M.D. The trauma service offered all the excitement and opportunity he could have asked for; with some highly preliminary numbers and a little fancy footwork, he and Marty convinced the hospital to fund a research fellowship in trauma, and suddenly there were three submariners instead of two. Nobody thought to question it: If the hospital was going to provide good trauma care, why not have a trauma research fellow? It made perfect sense.

Indeed, everything the trauma service did made perfect sense. In retrospect, that should have tipped off the opposition quicker than anything else.

It made excellent sense, for example, to issue red pagers to Mirean Coleman and Trent Lewis, the two senior social workers in the ER, and to incorporate them into the trauma team. Of course there needed to be someone to assist the family, bring them information, help them cope. It made equally good sense to have the senior doctor from the code room be the one who would eventually speak to the family to give them medical details and outlook. That way the family got a single, consistent story, not the interpretations of half a dozen different junior residents.

Indeed, it made excellent sense to staff the trauma team only with senior residents and attending-level staff; at least, it made sense until Marty started ordering the junior residents out of the code room. Until a patient was stable, he decreed, there would be nine and only nine people in the code room. He stayed outside himself, a coach on the sidelines, sometimes sending in a play or two, but in general letting the team do its work, uncluttered with junior—or senior—people.

The uproar was genteel, as befits physicians, but it was an uproar nevertheless. What did Eichelberger mean keeping residents out of the code room? This was a teaching hospital! How were junior people ever supposed to learn if they couldn't go in and watch?

Watch? Marty inquired. Not help? Just watch and listen? Heads nodded. Very well, Marty said. I agree. They should be allowed to watch and listen. Give me a couple of weeks to set it up.

Marty left the meeting, found McGinley. Shortly thereafter, color video cameras appeared in the corners of both code rooms, and microphones dangled from the ceilings. The sound and picture were piped into a tiny nurses' lounge behind the emergency room's main desk. Now when Marty threw junior residents out of the code room, he had a place to send them. He also had a highly diplomatic cover story. "It's so crowded in there you can't see anything," he would tell them. "Here you can see it all. That's why we put the system in."

There was a fringe benefit, too: They could videotape the trauma admissions that happened evenings and weekends, while Marty wasn't in the hospital. Then on Monday morning, he could watch them, like a coach watching his game films. More than once, the videotapes showed departures from the checklist, sometimes to the detriment of the child. Each such incident got mentioned to the offending party, and soon word got around: Eichelberger attends every trauma stat, either in person or electronically.

With the in-house systems working well enough to show off, McGinley turned his attention to the people who count most in a trauma system: the ambulance men in the field. Children's Hospital had a good working relationship with the District of Columbia Fire Department, which ran D.C.'s ambulance service. People from Children's, usually one of the emergency room docs, had always helped train new D.C. ambulance men on how to take care of injured kids. Now Tom McGinley delivered the lectures, and when he had aroused enough interest, he held the extra after-hours training sessions that the medics requested.

This was the real payoff from all Marty's trauma research in Philadelphia. The ambulance men had the medical training to understand when McGinley told them that, medically, children are very different from adults.

"They are not miniature adults," he would say, quoting pure Eichelberger. "The anatomy is not like an adult's. All the organs are different sizes. All the relationships are different. If you don't remember that, you can hurt the child."

For example, he would point out, a child's head is larger, in relation to the rest of the body. This makes children more vulnerable to head and neck injury. For another, a child has more body surface area, proportionately. That means they lose body heat faster. You have to think about that, think about ways to keep them warm.

The lectures contained example after example of special things that could go wrong with kids. The D.C. ambulance men were intrigued. McGinley got to know many of them on a first-name basis, and his newly acquired friends introduced him to other friends, paramedics who worked on the ambulances that served the wealthy D.C. suburbs.

Soon McGinley was giving his lecture in Bethesda, Fairfax, Chevy Chase, Arlington, Landover. The medics from the 'burbs ate up the new knowledge and wished aloud that there were a system for getting kids from their areas to Children's. But from outside the Washington beltway, it is a half-hour ride to Children's under the best of circumstances; during rush hour it's impossible. Wouldn't it be great if you guys had a helipad, the medics mused.

Yep, McGinley agreed, that would be great.

Back at the hospital, McGinley and Eichelberger set to work on a helipad. Washington Hospital Center, located adjacent to Children's, had a helipad for its MEDSTAR shock-trauma unit. McGinley and Eichelberger met with MEDSTAR director Howard Champion and received permission to use the helipad. They sent word to the suburban ambulance companies and, before long, a few injured kids began arriving by helicopter.

From the beginning, though, McGinley and Eichelberger knew that Children's would need its own helipad. The logistics were too complicated otherwise: On short notice, you had to summon a D.C. ambulance to move a patient from the MEDSTAR helipad to the Children's ER, and though the buildings were physically close, the layout of the streets made it a four- or five-minute trip. Sometimes that was too long; in really serious cases, the Children's trauma team had to "borrow" a resuscitation bay at MEDSTAR until the child was stable enough to move. Before long, McGinley started keeping extra packs of the special pediatric instruments at MEDSTAR; eventually one of MEDSTAR's trauma bays was unofficially reserved for the use of the Children's trauma team.

For a temporary solution, it worked well enough. In the few months he had been there, McGinley had already proved that Children's could attract more trauma cases, and that trauma cases were money-makers. His status changed from hired consultant to full-time employee. And his mission became, to the exclusion of nearly everything else, to get a helipad built for Children's Hospital.

He missed a few training sessions, and the paramedics complained. That was how Geraldine Pratch, RN, joined the submarine trauma staff.

Marty remembers the day he interviewed Gerry. She looked good on paper; she'd worked at Children's Hospital before, then had left to go back to school. Now she had a master's degree from the prestigious Johns Hopkins School of Public Health and was ready for new challenges.

"Do you know anything about trauma?" Marty asked.

Gerry's reply was offhand. "Only what I saw in Nam."

"Vietnam?" Marty's eyebrows went up. "What were you doing in Vietnam?"

"I was an army nurse for two years."

Marty offered her the job on the spot. She accepted on the spot. An army nurse would understand the realities of field medicine the way no civilian ever could. She would be able to deal with paramedics as an equal, with a kind of credibility that no master's degree could provide.

And Tom McGinley would have time to build his helipad.

McGinley had piloted fixed-wing aircraft, so he knew the basic rules of aerial navigation. One of the most basic rules is that to land someplace, you have to be able to find it.

The revolving aircraft beacon that McGinley installed on the roof of Children's Hospital made the place visible to pilots a hundred miles away. It got the hospital listed in all the FAA directories, and even commercial airline pilots were grateful for an additional reference point in the jumbled Washington night sky. The community of pilots is a small one, and word travels quickly among them. Almost overnight, Children's Hospital was a landmark for pilots. The beacon, expensive to install, provided some of the best, cheapest, and most enduring publicity Children's Hospital had ever received.

If they were going to run a helipad, it would be necessary to run a round-the-clock radio room, too. For one thing, the rules required it. For another, you had to have someone always available to alert the trauma team that something was on the way.

McGinley turned his attention to radio licenses, transmitters, antennas, wiring. Progress on the helipad slowed. The hospital had given its reluctant approval to the project, but when McGinley wasn't in there pushing, no one seemed anxious to keep things moving. McGinley and Eichelberger talked it over, and agreed that what they really needed was a good streetwise and traumawise administrator.

The person they recruited was Dennis Evans, a low-key but politically savvy refugee from Maryland's shock-trauma program. Evans had spent five years running the state program that organizes and trains paramedics in Maryland. Then, in one of the periodic management shakeups that have become a tradition at Shocktrauma, Evans found himself reassigned to a meaningless make-work job. At about the same time Eichelberger and McGinley started looking around, so did Dennis Evans.

With the arrival of an administrator, the trauma service, which still did not exist in theory, began to exist in fact—and visibly. An administrator meant there would be budgets, analyses of where the money would come from and where it would go; it meant there was suddenly someone in the hospital who spoke the administrator's language of goals and planning, and spoke it on behalf of a still-theoretical trauma service. It meant there was now someone with intimate knowledge of the Maryland EMS system, and with the connections to get Children's

Hospital officially designated as the pediatric trauma center not just for the nation's capital but for its Maryland suburbs. The Children's Hospital trauma program was about to start getting official recognition. The submarine was ready to surface.

Seven

Shortly after Mary Fallat left them, a social worker came to greet David and Patricia Myers. He helped them get little David registered and then took them to the code room, where David was being bundled for another ride, this time to the CAT scanner. "Remember," the social worker told them as they walked down the hall toward the code room, "be sure to sound upbeat and confident when you talk to him. If you sound upset, a child will pick that up, and he'll think you're mad at him."

As nurses and residents worked around them, Mr. and Mrs. Myers stood at the bedside for a long moment, saying nothing, looking at their son. Aside from a bright red scrape above his left eyebrow, he looked unhurt. He simply appeared to be asleep. A rigid plastic tube protruded from the left side of his mouth, and a flexible tube disappeared into his right nostril. Both tubes were held in place by two strips of white adhesive tape across his chin and upper lip; the strips of tape converged on both sides of his mouth, creating the effect of a clown's mask. His eyes were closed, and his chest heaved rhythmically as the respiratory technician squeezed the black bag attached to the airway tube.

David's left arm was securely taped to a gauze-covered board to protect his intravenous line, but the hand was still free, the fingers limp and curled. Tentatively, Mr. Myers grasped David's left hand. Then he gripped it more firmly. "Pookie," he said, leaning close to David's left ear. "Pookie, Mommy and Daddy are here. David, your Mommy and Daddy are here. David, can you squeeze my fingers?"

One of the residents looked up, then spoke. "He won't be able to squeeze your hand. We gave him medication to keep him still. But talk to him; he still may be able to hear you."

Mr. and Mrs. Myers looked at each other, then back at David. Then Mrs. Myers spoke: "David, you're in the hospital, but it's okay;

Mommy and Daddy are here. We love you, David, and we're gonna be right here with you." There were tears in her eyes as she spoke, but her voice remained perfectly calm.

◆ ◆ ◆

There are a few plastic chairs in the hallway outside the second-floor room that houses the CAT scanner, and as the bed containing David Myers rolled down the hallway, the social worker guided Mr. and Mrs. Myers toward the chairs. "X-rays," the social worker explained. "We can sit here, and when they're finished shooting, you can go in and be with him."

The three sat for several minutes, making small talk. When the social worker learned that Mr. Myers worked for the weather service, he inquired about next week's weather. Mr. Myers replied that his job was no longer directly involved in forecasting, and then launched into a lengthy and technical discussion of weather maps and weather patterns. The social worker listened, nodding politely, until Mrs. Myers finally broke in. "David," she said, "we don't understand all those isobars and millibars. The man just wants to know if it's going to rain."

The conversation lagged, which gave the social worker a chance to excuse himself. "Let me see how they're doing in there," he said.

◆ ◆ ◆

It is always crowded in the CAT scan control room. The room is precisely big enough for one technician and one radiologist, and even one more person constitutes a crowd. During a trauma admission, the place resembles a subway car during rush hour. The trauma coordinator, the surgical resident, the ICU resident, the charge nurse, and at least one other nurse nearly always accompany the patient to the CAT scanner. These individuals, the nucleus of the trauma team, are expected to be there, because until the CAT scans are complete, the checklist is not complete.

A dozen years ago, before there were CAT scanners in every hospital, it was routine to perform exploratory surgery on any patient suspected of having internal bleeding. This saved a great many lives, but it also left a great many accident victims with surgical scars that were, in hindsight, unnecessary.

The CAT scanner changed all that. With the ability to produce sharp, clear, three-dimensional pictures of a patient's insides, the laparotomy—the exploratory operation—suddenly became a rarity, limited to the occasional gunshot wound or stab wound where the patient is clearly losing blood rapidly.

The rest go to CAT scan, where a radiologist, not a surgeon, determines whether there are injuries requiring surgical repair. At Children's Hospital, the CAT scanner has worked so well that only 3 percent of all serious injuries result in abdominal surgery.

But in that rare instance where the CAT scanner shows serious internal bleeding, the trauma team has to be ready to head for the operating rooms at the other end of the second-floor hallway. So everyone crowds into the tiny CAT scan control room.

The social worker nudged a resident aside as he gently opened the door. "Anything?" he asked Mary Fallat.

"Nothing we didn't already suspect," the chief resident replied. "His brain is swelling pretty badly. We'll probably put in a bolt." A bolt is a device for monitoring the increased pressure that occurs inside the cranium when the brain swells. There are more technically precise names for it, but *bolt* is short and descriptive.

"Want me to explain anything to the parents?" asked the social worker.

"They already know about the bolt," Fallat replied. "I talked to them earlier. I'll stop and see them again when we're done in here."

♦ ♦ ♦

The intensive care unit is one floor up from X-ray, a four-minute trip including the wait for an elevator. The trauma team accompanied little David all the way through the double doors into the ICU and helped transfer the small body from the rolling bed onto the larger, and highly sophisticated, ICU bed. David's bed was bed number three, though the only way to figure that out was to count clockwise from the double doors. There were no such impersonal markings as numbers in this ICU; this, after all, was a children's hospital. On the wall behind David's new bed was a large cartoon of a floppy-eared rabbit.

David's parents stayed at the bedside during part of the trip. As they approached the ICU, the social worker drew them aside. "It's going to take them a while to get him set up," the social worker told them. "We'd just be in the way. Let me show you the waiting room."

Eight _____

Admitting little David Myers to the hospital generated a great deal of paper; everyone involved in the process had forms to complete. There were forms in the code room, forms in the admitting office, forms in the ECIC. David Hunter wrote steadily for ten minutes, pausing twice to answer the phone, and once more to phone the ambulance dispatcher, to verify the amount of time that had elapsed between the accident and little David's arrival at Children's. He snapped the multipart forms apart, deposited copies in all the proper pigeonholes and, after making minute adjustments to all the various radio channels on his control console, settled back to read his book. The day promised to be long and dull. The weather had turned progressively worse; an icy rain had joined the cold, blustery winds. It was not the sort of day when too many children would be outside.

Indeed, the next call did not come for more than an hour. An ambulance driver announced that they were on their way with a burn victim, a two-year-old girl with second- and third-degree burns of the face and arms. About 10 percent, the ambulance medic said.

Trauma medicine is, first and foremost, checklist medicine. On the battlefield, there is no time for learned consultations; there is only time to act. "Trauma stat. Burn. ER. Two minutes," Dave announced into the telephone. Seconds later, red pagers all over the hospital came to life.

In retrospect, Dave might have been able to forgo the full trauma stat for this particular case; the little girl had stumbled and fallen face first into an open space heater, the kind of heater that is, in fact, against the law for just such reasons. She had singed her hair and eyebrows, and she had minor burns on one cheek and on the tip of her nose. The real injury was to her left hand. Two fingers had gone directly into the red-hot grating, and in several small spots the flesh

61

was blackened, with red streaks showing through as the burned skin began to crack.

Even so, there was nothing even remotely life-threatening about her injuries, so the massed resources of the trauma team went largely unused. Within five minutes of the girl's arrival most of the trauma team members had excused themselves and gone back to their ordinary duties. No one complained; it was always better to err on the side of caution.

The little girl, of course, did not appreciate her good fortune. It did not matter to her that her mother had been close by when she stumbled and had pulled her away from the heater before any really serious injury occurred; nor did it matter that a trained ambulance crew had applied expert field dressings to her burns and had taken her to a hospital where there were specialists in the treatment of children's burns. Little Tonya Wallace knew only that she was in a great deal of pain, and her shrieks filled the hallway outside the code room and were plainly audible around the corner in the ECIC, where, less than ten minutes after the first call, Dave Hunter was being notified of yet another burn case on the way.

This time he was more cautious. The ambulance crew described second-degree burns to hands and forearms and estimated the burned area to be perhaps 10 percent of the child's body surface. The ambulance was a considerable distance away; ETA was ten minutes, the driver said.

Dave stood up and walked to the doorway of the ECIC. The doorway is surrounded by the square horseshoe of the emergency room nursing station desk, a constant beehive of activity. There are five telephones and two computer terminals on the bright blue countertop, and nearly all of them are almost always busy.

There is always at least one fully qualified pediatrician in the emergency room even on weekends. As Dave looked around the nursing station, he spotted Dr. Daniel Ochsenschlager, the chief ER pediatrician, who also happened to be the attending pediatrician for that day. Nobody tries to pronounce Dr. Ochsenschlager's last name; he is known by colleagues, subordinates, and patients alike simply as "Dan O." or, when more formality is required, "Dr. O."

Dr. O. is the perfect emergency room physician; nothing upsets him. In all his years of managing the constant bedlam of an emergency room, he has never screamed at anyone, never raised his voice at all, except to be heard over the normal din of the ER. Rumor has it that he has gotten angry on occasion, but few people have actually seen it happen. His even temper is legendary, and his relaxed, informal demeanor has helped calm the hysteria of literally thousands of anxious parents.

◆ ◆ ◆

Dave caught Dr. O.'s eye. "Another burn coming," Dave announced, raising his voice so Dr. O. could hear him. "Second-degree, ten percent. Want me to call another code?"

Dr. O. shook his head. "Nah," he said, smiling. "Let's look at him first." The last one had been borderline; if the trauma team got summoned for enough borderline cases, there would be grumbling. And if the child arrived in much worse shape than expected, they could always call a trauma stat right from the examining room.

Dan O. met the ambulance crew at the sliding glass doors, and directed them into the second code room. It had the advantage of being a one-bed room; the examining rooms down the hall all had multiple beds, separated only by thin curtains. A young burn victim's cries would only upset the children in adjacent beds. And if he did have to call a trauma stat, Dr. O. wanted the child in the right place.

The boy was about four, the age at which many children are unbearably cute, but this child, whose name was Richard, had an unkempt look about him. His sandy hair was ragged and oily; his face was smudged and grimy, as were his bare feet. Both his hands and forearms were bright red, and he held them slightly away from his body.

But he wasn't crying.

"Hi, Richard, my name is Dan O."

"Hi." Richard's reply was polite but distant. He wouldn't look directly at Dr. O.

"What happened to your hands?"

"I . . . burned them in hot water."

"He fell," a female voice behind Dan O. said. "He fell forward into a tub of hot water." Dr. O. looked around and saw a woman who looked as unkempt and unwashed as the boy.

Dr. O. smiled. "Are you Richard's mother?" he asked. The woman nodded. "This doesn't look too bad," Dr. O. continued, "but I want to check him over just to be sure. If you want to have a seat out in the hall, I'll come get you as soon as I'm done." This, too, was unusual: When children are not seriously hurt, the parents usually stay right at their side; it helps keep the children calm. Something was wrong here, though: Richard was too calm already. Dan had an uncomfortable feeling about the case.

"Richard," he said, turning back to the boy on the examining table, "I need to look at your arms for a minute. Which one should I do first?" Richard lifted the left arm slightly; it was the one closest to Dr. O.

Gently, he touched the reddened flesh. Richard winced and softly said "owww," but he did not draw his arm away. Dan checked both sides of the arm, then checked the other arm. No blisters were forming, which was a good sign. He instructed a nurse to apply an ointment to the hands and arms; the ointment contained a mild anesthetic, which would ease the sting. Richard's burns were about the caliber of a medium-bad sunburn. He'd been fortunate.

Or perhaps *lucky* was not the right word. The burns extended midway up the boy's forearms, and there was a clear, straight demarcation line between the reddened area and the white skin above it. There were no splash marks above the burned area.

Working slowly, methodically, Dr. O. began an examination of the boy's body. The bottoms of the boy's feet were rough and callused, a sign that he went barefoot a great deal. The little toe on the right foot was bent at an odd angle, but when Dr. O. manipulated each of the toes in turn, the boy made no sign that anything hurt. It looked as though the toe had been broken at some previous time and had healed without being properly splinted.

The boy was clad in shorts and a T-shirt, unusual garb considering the weather outside. With a pair of shovel-nosed scissors, Dr. O. cut away the T-shirt so he could examine the rest of the boy's upper body. The pale flesh was grimy, and there were four small scars, two old ones down low on the boy's back and two newer ones, just below Richard's left nipple. The scars were round, surfaced with the tough, wrinkled white flesh that grows when a burn heals. Each of the scars was about the diameter of a pencil eraser—or a lit cigarette.

"I'm going to admit him," Dr. O. said to the nurse in the room with him. "You're in charge for a minute; I'll be right back." He strode briskly out of the code room, smiled at Richard's mother as he walked past her, but continued down the hallway to the nursing station and made two right turns, into the ECIC, where the ambulance medic was busy filling out forms. "What can you tell me about Richard?" he asked the medic.

"Bad place," the medic said. "Filthy. Smells. Mom made the call. Boyfriend was there, but he stayed in the other room while we were there. Mom said the kid fell in the tub. You see any splash marks?"

Dan O. shook his head. "Thanks," he said. He walked slowly back to where Richard's mother was sitting, alone. He sat down next to her, smiling as always. "Is your husband here?" he asked.

"He's not my husband," the woman said. "He's my fiancé. He had to go to work."

Dan smiled. "I see. Well, I'm sure you'll want to call him. Richard's going to be okay. The burns are serious, but they're not too deep, and I don't think there'll be any permanent damage."

Dan chose his next words very carefully. "But with a case like this you can't be too careful, so I want to admit him to the burn unit at least until tomorrow, so we can keep an eye on him." The woman nodded. Dan paused a moment, then continued. "There is one other issue you need to know about, and that is the . . . unusual nature of Richard's burns. Usually when a child falls into some hot liquid, there are splash marks, but Richard has no splash marks. We've had cases like that in the past where it turned out the injuries were not accidental, so I'm going to ask our Division of Child Protection to take a look at Richard, just to make sure everything's okay."

Still smiling, Dan excused himself and headed back to the nursing station to start the necessary paperwork.

The doctors and nurses who work in the emergency room see lots of cases like this, and the one universal rule they follow is: Avoid passing judgment. Avoid confrontations. Protect the kid, but suppress the anger that wells up at the sight of a four-year-old who clearly has been tortured.

The first form that Dan O. filled out was a referral to the hospital's Division of Child Protection.

Nine

Patricia and David Myers spent a long, fidgety time in the waiting room outside the Intensive Care Unit. It was a longer wait than they expected. Things stayed busy around ICU bed number three for the next two hours as several teams of specialists and nurses prepared little David for his convalescence.

As David was being lifted onto the ICU bed, the anesthesiologist was already making settings on the mechanical respirator that sat at the head of the bed. As soon as David was properly positioned in the bed, the respiratory technician removed the black bag from David's airway tube and replaced it with the respirator hose.

David might conceivably have been able to breathe on his own, but the odds were great he wouldn't have done it well enough to get oxygen to his injured brain. David's chest X-ray showed dark spots in the upper half of his lungs. The dark spots were bruises, caused by the impact of the car. The bruised lung tissue would be less efficient at moving oxygen into the blood, and even though no ribs were broken, David would have found it painful to breathe on his own, so he would have breathed only when he couldn't avoid it.

The respirator, by contrast, inflated his lungs a precise twenty-one times per minute and, more important, it kept pressure in the lungs all the time, never letting them deflate completely. This "positive end expiratory pressure," called PEEP for short, is part of the standard treatment for bruised lungs and for head injuries that involve brain swelling. It forces more oxygen into the blood than would normally be there, in the hope that enough of it will get through to the brain to keep that organ from dying.

So even though the main threat to David's life was his swollen brain, the main threat to the brain at the moment was his damaged lungs. The anesthesiologist and respiratory tech watched the respirator for several minutes and ordered an immediate blood sample to be sent to the lab, to reassure themselves that David's blood was 100 percent saturated with oxygen.

Once the anesthesiology team was finished, they stepped away from the bedside and let the neurosurgery resident take over. With the lungs under control, it was time to do whatever could be done for the other potentially lethal problem, the high pressure inside David's skull.

Moving around to the head of the bed, the neurosurgeon swabbed some brown antiseptic over David's short hair, then picked up a disposable razor and began to shave away the hair from the right side of the boy's head. He went over the area twice to make sure the skin was perfectly smooth, then wiped it several times with antiseptic towels. Once satisfied that every trace of hair was gone, the neurosurgeon began draping sterile coverings over all exposed surfaces, including David's upper body. Then, breaking open a sterile package, he took out a surgical drape and aligned it over David's head so that only the newly created bald spot showed.

"Ready?" the neurosurgeon asked the ICU nurse who'd been assigned to David. She nodded, handing the surgeon a pack of sterile gloves and breaking another open for herself.

First, the neurosurgeon injected epinephrine—Adrenalin—into the bare skin of David's scalp. This powerful stimulant caused the tiny blood vessels in the scalp to contract tightly, so that, a moment later, when the scalpel parted the skin, the white fat below showed for several seconds before the blood began to ooze. Working swiftly but carefully, the surgeon sliced downward until he could see gleaming bright bone. He held the scalpel out to the nurse, who took it from his hand and replaced it with a pair of special forceps designed for spreading instead of clamping. The surgeon maneuvered the end of the spreader into the incision, then squeezed the handle. Tiny stainless-steel fingers grasped both sides of the surgical wound, spreading it wide and exposing a small diamond of skull below. "Okay, let me have the craniotome," he said to the nurse.

A craniotome looks a great deal like the sort of hand drill you'd find in a hardware store. The principal difference is that a craniotome is all stainless steel and costs several hundred dollars. And it has a special drill-bit assembly that disengages as soon as the skull has been penetrated. The neurosurgeon maneuvered the bit against David's skull, leaned forward to put pressure on the drill, and began turning the crank. Shreds of bone filled the incision, and the nurse sprayed sterile water into the wound, both to keep the drilling site cool and to wash away the bone fragments. The maneuver took only a few seconds; the bit disengaged with a sharp click, and the neurosurgeon withdrew the craniotome. The nurse rinsed the wound one final time, and the surgeon got his first look at the dura, the leathery sac that encases the brain.

Half an hour earlier, while the CAT scanner was busy looking inside David's abdomen for signs of internal bleeding, the neurosurgeon had been intently studying the images of the inside of David's head. He knew the worst damage was on the right side; the fact that David's right pupil was larger than the left told him that. The CAT scans told him the details. Inside the right hemisphere, the ventricle —a long narrow cistern of spinal fluid—was squeezed almost completely shut. The pressure in the right side of David's brain was dangerously high.

Only a few things can be done to relieve pressure inside the head. One is to give the patient a powerful diuretic, forcing the kidneys to make lots of urine, dehydrating the rest of the system, including the brain. The brain contains a great deal of liquid; removing some of it will give the brain more room to swell, keeping the pressure down.

But you can give only so much diuretic without damaging other parts of the body. The ventilator can help minimize the damage caused by brain swelling, but that only helps for so long. If the swelling is too great, the blood supply is completely choked off, and the brain dies.

A ventriculostomy serves two purposes. The first is to allow precise measurement of the pressure inside the head. The second is to allow drainage of spinal fluid when the pressure gets too high. The surgeon uses the term *ventriculostomy* only when writing in the medical record; in conversation, the procedure is called "putting in a bolt."

It is more than an analogy. The stainless steel intracranial pressure monitor has self-tapping threads; after making a tiny pinprick in the tough dura, the neurosurgeon fitted the small device against the edge of the hole and began to twist. The slender stainless steel tube protruding from the inside of the bolt had been precisely measured, so that when the bolt was screwed snugly against David's skull, the hollow tip of the device rested precisely in the center of David's right ventricle. A small amount of spinal fluid spurted out the top of the bolt before the flow eased to a steady dribble.

The neurosurgeon attached a wire to the top of the bolt and, at the bedside, an orange wave form jumped crazily on an oscilloscope screen, then settled into a steady pattern that mimicked David's heartbeat. Beside the wave form, numbers flashed rapidly on the screen, then stabilized at 18. The pressure in David's head was safely low now. The neurosurgeon carefully stitched the scalp into place around the bolt, then applied sterile dressings to the wound. Finally, he put a protective cover over the entire assembly and wrapped adhesive tape around that, securing it to the top of David's head.

The ICP monitor stayed steady at 18. That was not good, but it was acceptable. As long as the intracranial pressure stayed less than the blood pressure in David's arteries, his heart would have no problem forcing blood through the vessels of his brain. The neurosurgeon watched the monitor as he jotted notes on David's chart. David was safe for the moment but would need constant watching. Even before the neurosurgeon left the bedside, the pressure reading had advanced to 19.

With David's lungs and head accounted for, the two orthopedic residents who had been lounging nearby sauntered over to the bedside. Now it was their turn. Broken bones are seldom fatal, so on the trauma checklist of priorities, they usually come last.

Pediatric orthopedics is a happy specialty. The standard joke is that if you can get the two ends of a broken bone anywhere in the same room, they will grow together and align themselves. There is truth, however exaggerated, in the saying; children's bones, because they are still growing, have the ability to heal and reshape themselves so that, in some cases, it becomes difficult after a few years to tell that there was ever a fracture.

But a growing bone also presents problems. In the process of knitting itself back together, a broken bone grows faster than an unbroken one. Years ago, pediatric orthopedic surgeons learned the hard way that if they set a child's broken leg the same way they would an adult's, that leg would grow to be longer than the other one. The disability was usually small, often not noticeable by anyone except the child, but in some cases the surgeon was later required to remove a chunk of the leg bone to bring the legs back to their proper alignment.

The solution to this problem turned out to be ridiculously simple: Don't set a broken femur. Let the two jagged ends overlap. Hang the broken leg in traction to keep it immobile, and in about three weeks the overlapping bones will fuse tightly enough together to allow the leg to be put in a cast. Six more weeks and the child can begin to walk on the leg. Six months later, if you X-ray the leg, you will see that the excess bone around the junction has begun to dissolve away, leaving the child with a femur that is not only the correct length but probably stronger than the original. Pediatric orthopods speak almost worshipfully of Mother Nature's methods and abilities.

But for all the beauty of a properly healed femur, the process of getting it there, as managed by the orthopedic surgeon, is unlovely. David had already received a small dose of morphine before the neurosurgeon performed his procedure; now, just to be safe, the ortho-pods gave David a little more. Then they went to work inserting stainless steel pins into both sides of each of his thighs, just above the knees. This involved the use of another instrument that brought to mind the neurosurgeon's craniotome. Each of the pins was threaded on one end. The other end went into the chuck of the hand drill, a little incision was made through the fleshy part of the leg, and the pin, held in the hand drill, was threaded through the wound until the screw threads touched the bone. Then, while one resident held the leg still, the other one turned the crank on the drill until the screw threads cut deeply into the bone, making a tight bond.

When the pins were securely in place on both sides of each leg, the two surgeons began arranging a traction apparatus over the bed. First they attached a central overhead frame to both ends of the bed; from this they hung crossbars with pulleys and threaded ropes through the pulleys. They attached ropes to the pins protruding from David's legs and hung bags of sand on the other ends, to provide a constant pull on the ropes. They tinkered and adjusted until David's thighs were approximately vertical. Then they attached two more ropes to soft fleece-lined stirrups, designed to hold the calves of David's legs hori-zontal, at ninety-degree angles to the thighs. This ninety-ninety trac-tion, orthopods long ago learned, is the best position for a patient with a broken femur.

The two residents conferred over David's X-rays a while longer. The right leg would be the toughest, they agreed. That fracture was very near the hipbone, and they weren't sure, but it looked as if there might have been a chip of bone knocked out of the hip joint as well. That one might eventually need surgery, but there were, the residents knew, other problems to sort out first. The left leg would be a breeze. Simple fracture, two-thirds of the way down the leg. It would heal with no problem.

David's third fracture, which had gone virtually unnoticed during his admission, was his left collarbone. The X-rays showed it, and the orthopedic residents duly noted its presence on David's chart, but they did nothing except order a folded towel to be placed under David's right shoulder to brace the area. All you can do for a fractured clavicle is immobilize it, and David was already immobile. Besides, both ends of the clavicle were well within the same room; they would heal just fine.

◆ ◆ ◆

It was another half hour before David's parents finally came in. Once she had finished assisting all the various specialists with their procedures, David's nurse had to go through her own set of procedures. Working quietly, methodically, she untangled the spaghetti mound of IV tubing that had accumulated near the head of David's bed. One by one she identified each line, tabbed it with adhesive tape, and marked it with a pen so she'd be able to identify it quickly next time, ran her hands along the full length of it to make sure it wasn't kinked, carefully coiled up the excess tubing, and secured each coil with adhesive tape.

She drew a fresh blood sample, maneuvered a rectal thermometer into place and, when it showed David's body temperature to be a little cool, put a blanket over his torso. She checked the Foley catheter that drained into a bag on the side of the bed and made a note of David's urine output. She checked the tube in David's nose. She applied antibacterial ointment to the one visible wound above his left eye. She listened to his heart and lungs with her stethoscope; gently squeezed his thumbnail, and noted how long it took to turn pink again; felt for pulses in both feet, and shone her flashlight into both his eyes.

Finally, when she was satisfied that her patient was ready, she walked to the waiting room, introduced herself to David's parents, and escorted them to his bedside. It was 9:30 P.M., nearly six hours after the accident.

A full-size bed makes a small patient look even smaller. With his legs dangling in the air, David took up only a quarter of the bed's surface, near the head. At the foot of the bed, safe from any movement by the patient, lay an orange plastic dishpan containing several dozen hypodermic syringes, each in a sterile plastic container; a clipboard containing a sheet for the nurse's notes; an electronic thermometer; a package of tissues; and a folded bedsheet. Just beyond the head of the bed, a boxlike respirator gave off a steady *hiss-click, hiss-click,* as it breathed for David. Out of the respirator snaked a pair of long blue hoses that merged together in a Y-shaped manifold connected to the airway tube in David's mouth.

Intravenous lines sprouted from David's neck, from his groin, and from both arms. The tangle of tubing led in two directions: Some of the tubes were connected to pale blue IV pump boxes with flashing lights; the remaining tubes and wires ended at an electronic manifold connector that was in turn connected to the electronic bedside monitor, whose screen displayed, in vivid orange, a series of wave forms and numbers. In the center of this high-tech jumble, David lay perfectly still, chest heaving rhythmically, eyes closed, looking unconcernedly, peacefully asleep.

"David," the nurse announced in a voice that was not loud but carried. "David, guess what. Your mom and dad are here." She motioned them to the right side of the bed, which was relatively free of medical debris.

You can say only so much to an unconscious person. Mr. and Mrs. Myers stood close to their son's bedside and made small talk for a while. Finally, they just stood quietly. Mrs. Myers held David's hand while Mr. Myers stroked his shoulder.

They talked to the nurse a great deal. Both of them, but especially Mr. Myers, were interested in every minute detail of David's treatment. In response to various questions, the nurse explained to them that there would be no casts on David's legs for several weeks. She explained why it was important to tape every tube securely into place, especially the one that extended into David's brain. She gave them a guided tour of all David's tubes and showed them the corresponding numbers on the monitor screen. She agreed that the scrape over David's eye would probably leave a scar. She told them that although

David was unconscious and paralyzed with drugs, he might well be able to hear them, and that he could certainly feel their touch. They should talk to him and touch him as much as they wanted. Kids do better, she said, when you talk to them and touch them a lot.

Ten

Not long after the helipad was completed, Tom McGinley turned in his resignation. He'd accomplished the things he'd come there to do, he told Dr. Eichelberger, and now it was time to look for something else. With the trauma program firmly established, he said, Eichelberger no longer needed a submarine pilot. He needed a diplomat, and that was out of McGinley's line. After the requisite exit interviews and farewell parties, McGinley packed his bags and headed for Pittsburgh. The care and feeding of the trauma program fell to Dennis Evans.

Evans was hired to be an administrator, to build and supervise a professional staff that would make sure the trauma system always worked, and worked well. That meant a nearly continuous problem-solving operation, making sure all the proper supplies were in the right places, making sure all the paperwork was filled out correctly, making sure all the designated trauma team members always got to the code rooms within the specified number of minutes—watching to make sure things got done right, and when they didn't, finding out why and fixing the problem.

After McGinley announced his resignation, Evans and Eichelberger spent several lengthy sessions trying to decide where to look for the next trauma coordinator. They needed someone who could get along well with the paramedics in the field, and they needed someone who could monitor the quality of care given inside the hospital. If possible, they needed someone who could do all that without upsetting the fine political balance on which the trauma program perched.

It was a head scratcher. Evans went over and over his mental list of possibilities, trying to figure out whom he would call first, when he got an unexpected phone call from one of the hospital's assistant nursing directors, Heidi Zwick. She had heard about a vacancy, she told Evans, and she would like to buy him a cup of coffee and talk about it.

The cup of coffee became two cups, then three, and at quitting time they were still chatting. As one of the assistant nursing directors, Heidi was already a member of the trauma stat team, the member who stood just outside the door, made sure only the authorized people got in, coordinated the activities and filled out all the forms for the "outer core" team, and stood near a telephone to relay orders, consultation requests, lab results, and the like. Heidi had recently been chosen Employee of the Year by the hospital's employee relations committee. That was a plus; anyone that well known and well liked would be welcome in the corps of medical diplomats Evans needed so desperately.

But in addition to that, Evans learned, she had experience. She'd stood watch during trauma stats for three and a half years; for the three and a half years before that, she'd been the charge nurse in the emergency room on the evening shift, traditionally the busiest shift. She had been there when Eichelberger and McGinley first proposed using a trauma protocol, and she had seen the dramatic improvements that had followed. She'd also worked in the burn unit, the cardiology unit, and the intensive care unit. It was as though her entire career had been focused around the care of injured or acutely ill children.

And she wanted the job McGinley was vacating.

This, Evans realized, was not an opportunity to be missed. There were formalities, of course, job postings and personnel procedures to follow, but it was tough to imagine a candidate who could match or beat those credentials. Heidi had herself a new job.

For Heidi's part, her single request to Evans was, "Don't bore me." Every job she'd had before, she told him, had eventually become just another routine. When that happened, she got restless. Usually that meant another job. Evans promised not to bore her.

After three years on the job, Heidi agrees that she has never been bored. Many other adjectives—*frustrated, bemused, angry, fatigued*—would apply on occasion, but not *bored*. The job she took over from Tom McGinley has changed radically; after all, there are no more helipads to build. She inherited a trauma system that was already in place. Her job is not to build but to refine.

Evans, immersed in budgets and revenue projections, immediately handed over his trouble-shooting responsibilities to Heidi. After standing outside the code room for three and a half years, Heidi knew the trauma protocols and checklists by heart, and she knew all the

players by their first names. If something didn't go exactly as planned
—someone missed a step in the trauma ballet—Heidi was in a position
to notice and to make casual mention of it. Casual mention by Heidi
Zwick was generally more low-key than casual mention by Marty
Eichelberger; with Heidi doing the confronting, tensions diminished
between the unofficial trauma service and the official departments and
services.

Heidi carried one of the red pagers, of course, and whenever the
"trauma stat" alarm sounded, she headed for the code room, not to
participate in the ballet but to watch with a critical eye, as Marty had
always done. In the beginning, Marty always came, too, but with
Heidi there as his surrogate, he soon began to stay away. Now it was
Heidi who occasionally offered quiet suggestions about this problem
or that procedure. They were suggestions, not instructions, but it was
clear to the trauma team that a suggestion from Heidi, if ignored,
could result in a visit from Marty.

Heidi took over reviewing Marty's "game films," the videotapes of
admissions on evenings and weekends. If she spotted things that
needed mentioning to some member of the trauma team, she mentioned them. If the trauma team member told her to go to hell, she
mentioned it to Marty. It seldom happened twice.

Still, with Heidi established as keeper of the protocols, life got more
relaxed. Heidi was a strong advocate of the use of common sense. The
beauty of a trauma protocol is that the most unimaginative physician
in the world, if he follows the checklist, will have consistently good
results. But the physicians who work on the Children's Hospital
trauma team are no dullards; this, in Heidi's view, left room for
occasional departures from protocol. All she demanded was that the
exceptions make sense.

Always consider the "mechanism of injury," she would tell people.
Look at the circumstances of the accident. If a child has had a foot
cut off by a lawnmower, don't waste time on the part of the protocol
that looks for broken necks. If it's a burn case, don't spend time trying
to diagnose internal injuries. Sometimes it makes sense to depart from
the protocol; but *don't be wrong.* Be sure of what you're doing. If
you're not 100 percent sure, then follow the protocol and you'll never
get into trouble.

Heidi's troubleshooting role began to take on many of the characteristics of a quality-assurance coordinator. Quality assurance is big in hospitals these days; for one thing, accrediting agencies require aggressive Q-A programs. For another, monitoring the quality of care helps hospitals keep from getting sued, by reducing screwups to a minimum.

Physicians did considerable squirming, and a significant amount of yelling, when the concept of quality review was first advanced. Quality medical care is a subjective thing, they insisted; you can't measure the quality of medical care. They were right. Statistics can't measure quality.

But statistics can, it seems, measure the *absence* of quality. Quality assurance approaches the problem from that direction, asking not how good a physician is but rather how bad he is.

Or how potentially bad he is. The Q-A screening process does not produce answers, only more questions. It identifies the cases in which a patient did not progress according to normal expectations. For example, if a patient has surgery on Tuesday, and then requires two additional units of blood on Wednesday, or if the patient is unexpectedly taken back to the operating room on Thursday, a Q-A eyebrow will go up. It could simply be that the patient was very sick to begin with and started to go sour on them. Most Q-A "hits," when investigated, turn out to be false alarms.

But about 9 percent are real. An unplanned return to the OR occasionally means that the surgeon did something wrong and had to go back and do it over. If you investigate all unplanned returns to the OR, you will follow a lot of false leads, but you will also learn which surgeons are good—or more precisely, which ones are not.

A case that gets caught in the Q-A screen will be put on a list, to be discussed at the monthly meeting called the mortality and morbidity conference. Medical people, with their love of abbreviations, call it M and M rounds. At M and M rounds, cases that varied from the norm are reviewed by a group of physicians and Q-A people. Where the cause of the variation is determined to be incorrect or inadequate care, the responsible physician is invited to explain himself. A physician invited to explain himself often enough can find himself invited to practice medicine elsewhere. Hospitals pay breathtaking sums for malpractice insurance as it is; physicians who regularly produce potential lawsuits are increasingly unwelcome.

Marty Eichelberger was a Q-A nut long before he heard the term *Q-A*. He had spent the last few years doing curbside Q-A outside the code room or in front of a video screen. His standard was a simple one: Every kid that comes in the door will get the same treatment that Marty would expect for Todd and Lindsay Eichelberger. That was why there were protocols in the code room. When he learned that quality-assurance review could produce hard numbers, he became instantly enthusiastic about the idea. Numbers, Marty knew, were a trauma surgeon's ultimate source of power. The job of trauma coordinator rapidly became oriented around an aggressive Q-A screening process.

◆ ◆ ◆

Nobody would ever accuse Heidi Zwick of being a "morning person." She had always enjoyed working evening shifts, and gave it up only because evening work makes for a boring social life. But one of the disadvantages of being on the day shift was having to be at work before the 7:00 A.M. shift change. The hours of a trauma coordinator are more flexible. There are still days when Heidi arrives before seven, but now there are also days when she can wait until eight, sometimes even nine.

The luxury of this goes beyond the ability to sleep late. Rush hour in Washington, D.C., is one of the worst anywhere. Between 6:00 A.M. and 9:00 A.M. the population of the District of Columbia triples, and most of the increase arrives in cars. On some roads the traffic begins to back up at 5:30 A.M. By seven, every expressway is clogged to a crawl, an event so routine that the traffic reports don't even mention it. By eight, the worst is over, and by nine the streets have returned almost to normal. The most coveted jobs in Washington are the ones that start at nine.

Heidi uses a back route that usually begins to clear by eight, making the drive in from Bethesda last only about half an hour. On this particular Monday morning, traffic had been unusually light, and Heidi pulled her bright red sports car into the employee parking lot shortly after 8:15. Mondays were catch-up days: An entire weekend's worth of trauma cases would be awaiting review.

Heidi's office is on the first floor, but her first stop of the morning is always on the second floor, at the bank of huge coffee urns in the hospital cafeteria. She filled a gigantic Styrofoam cup, the one that costs sixty cents even with the employee discount. She loaded it up with two dollops of cream and three packets of sugar, clamped a plastic lid on it, paid the cashier, and trudged off toward her office. The admissions roster, as always, was waiting on her desk. No matter how early she got there, it was always waiting for her. It was a printout of all admissions to the hospital for the twenty-four hours that ended at midnight. Today there were three of them; one each for Friday, Saturday, and Sunday. Heidi peeled back the lid from her coffee cup, took a sip, and started on Friday's report.

Deciphering the computer printouts is an art in itself. Not every emergency admission qualifies as a trauma case; there are burns, and asthma cases, babies with diarrhea so severe that they require hospitalization, and an amazing variety of other problems and conditions. The computer provides only scant space for a description of the patient's problem, so the information is always abbreviated. Some of the abbreviations are obvious, like MVA for "motor vehicle accident," and occasionally she even sees the word "trauma" on the printout. Others, like "resp depres" could mean anything, including respiratory depression secondary to being hit by a car.

One of the entries on the Friday printout listed "PTX" as the reason for admission. Heidi reached for a blank index card. Pneumothorax does occur for reasons other than traumatic injury, but only rarely. At the top of the card, Heidi carefully copied the name "Jackson, Michael," and was already copying the age before she did a double take and smiled at the name. She took another sip of coffee. It was still very early in the morning.

By 9:30 she had a small stack of cards filled out and sorted according to what part of the hospital the patient was in. The top card on the stack read "Myers, David," and "ICU." She tossed the empty coffee cup in the trash can, pulled on the universal symbol of authority in a hospital—a white lab coat—and started on her rounds.

◆ ◆ ◆

As soon as Heidi walked through the double doors and into the intensive care unit, she could tell which case was David Myers. Orthopedic traction gear is visible from a great distance; little David was surrounded by enough girders, ropes, and pulleys for a medium-size trapeze act. There might as well have been a flag waving over bed number three.

Sitting in a plastic chair at the foot of the bed, an ICU nurse was busy writing. On the right side of the bed, Heidi saw a petite, attractive woman, sitting half-perched on a shiny stool. Even at a distance, the woman looked exhausted. Small wonder, Heidi thought, if she's been here since yesterday afternoon. With a nod of greeting to the nurse, Heidi walked around and stood beside Mrs. Myers.

"Hi," she said without preamble. "I'm Heidi. I'm the trauma coordinator. Are you Mrs. Myers?" The woman nodded. Heidi turned and took her first close look at little David. "God, what a cute kid," she murmured. "How's he doing?" she asked, not taking her eyes off the boy.

"He had a pretty rough night," Mrs. Myers answered, too tired to see the irony in being asked to give the trauma coordinator a medical briefing. In fact, Heidi already knew how David was doing; the question was designed more to see how David's mother was doing. "His blood pressure kept going down, and the pressure inside his head kept going up, but he's been better for the last few hours." She spoke slowly; her voice sounded tired, but the words were reasoned, calm, appropriate. Mothers who are about to become hysterical have a certain quiver in their voices, and a sort of staccato rush to their words. Their voices move to a higher pitch, and their answers tend to ramble. Conversely, mothers who are dangerously depressed speak only reluctantly, and without any inflection at all. Mrs. Myers's words had none of those warning signs, but they carried such pain and fatigue that Heidi winced mentally. Still, she listened politely as Mrs. Myers continued. "Last night they were afraid we might lose him," she said, "but just a little while ago Dr. Karmy-Jones told us that since he had gotten through the night okay, his chances are better now."

"Karmy-Jones is taking care of David?" Heidi asked. Mrs. Myers nodded. "That's good news." She let her voice drop to a conspiratorial whisper. "Kay-Jay is good. He's very good. One of the best." She saw Mrs. Myers brighten visibly. "I gotta go," she said. "I just stopped by to say hello. I'll be in and out; if you have any problems or questions about David, or about anything, let me know." She took one last look at David. "He sure is cute," she said again. Then she headed for the nursing desk. Heidi considers herself to be a very tough cookie, as indeed anyone who has spent a decade around badly hurt children must be. But there was something contagious about Mrs. Myers's grief, and Heidi was happy to retreat to the detached objectivity of

David's medical record. Most cases at Children's Hospital have happy endings, but a predictable few do not. Over time, the tragedies mount up; sooner or later they come out. Heidi once surprised even herself by bursting into tears in a movie theater during the sad part of *Terms of Endearment.* Worse, she permanently frightened away her date by continuing to cry for the next four hours. When she thought about it later, she realized that the tragedy in the movie had unleashed four or five years' worth of similar tragedies that she had witnessed or taken part in but had kept bottled up inside. When she tells the story now, Heidi shrugs; that sort of thing happens. It goes with the territory. You can't work in a hospital if you can't handle bad news sometimes. Still, the kid really was cute.

Heidi dragged an empty chair up to the nursing desk and opened David's medical record. He'd been in the hospital less than twenty-four hours, and already the chart was two dozen pages long. Heidi spends a good part of every day at nursing stations, reading medical records. Many quality-assurance programs are retrospective; the review takes place only after the patient is discharged. This is a definite benefit to future patients, but it can be tough on the ones who help identify the problems. On the trauma service, the Todd-and-Lindsay rule prevails: *Every* kid gets the care that Marty's own kids would get. That means daily review of every chart to identify any potential problems and fix them before they materialize.

As she leafed through the chart, Heidi paused occasionally to write on her index card. In cramped but legible handwriting, she copied the names of David's mother and father, their address and phone number. She carefully noted each of David's injuries, and made a list of the various specialists who had been called in for consultation on each of the injuries. She leafed through the chart, reading the handwritten notes by each of the specialists. She jotted down blood-pressure figures and lab test results, noted the fluctuations in David's intracranial pressure readings, and copied the time of admission from the chrono-logical event sheet the emergency room nurse had filled out. She turned a page and paused: The record of the ambulance crew showed that the accident happened nearly an hour before David got to the hospital. That was a long time, longer than one would expect. She made a note on her card. That was worth a phone call to the ambulance service's medical director. There was probably a perfectly good explanation, but it was Heidi's job to check. The Todd-and-Lindsay rule required it.

Heidi spent another ten minutes with little David's chart; it was already voluminous; hospitals require that all medical care be documented in excruciating detail. Some charts grow so huge that they have to be divided into several volumes.

Then, one by one, she went over the charts of the three other trauma cases currently in the ICU. Two had come in over the weekend. One had internal injuries from a fall; the other had suffered head injuries in a car accident. Children, especially small children, are prone to head injuries because the head is bigger, in proportion to body size, than in an adolescent or an adult. Happily, children seem to tolerate head injuries better than adults. As she reviewed the child's chart, Heidi was pleased to note signs of improvement; the child had begun to show purposeful movement. Usually, when that happened, they opened their eyes within another day or two.

The third chart was more grim; another unrestrained small child in another car accident. Another head injury, but this one was very, very severe. The child had been comatose for several days; the CAT scans showed severe brain damage. The child was not expected to survive. Heidi shook her head; it was never easy to watch a child die. Then she duly noted the child's continuing deterioration on her index card.

She had a fourth index card, but the patient was no longer to be found in the ICU. "Where'd Teresa go?" Heidi asked a nurse at the ICU main desk.

"IMCU. Yesterday." The Intermediate Care Unit is one step down from the ICU. It is a place for children who are no longer sick enough for an intensive care environment, but not yet ready for a general care bed. The proportion of nurses to patients is high; kids who still need special care go to the IMCU. Teresa would certainly need a lot of attention.

Teresa and her brother Tom had arrived in the same ambulance, the previous Thursday afternoon. Both had multiple injuries, including the near-inevitable head injury.

Tom had not survived. Nor had their mother, who was driving the children home from school when her car was hit broadside and crushed by a dump truck. Teresa, who was in the back seat, was not wearing a seat belt and was thrown against the door, where her head smashed into the door handle, fracturing her skull and mercifully knocking her unconscious.

In the front seat, both Tom and his mother were wearing seat belts, but the belts were scant protection against twelve tons of dump truck. The truck scooted the car across the street like a toy, mashed it up against a stone retaining wall and, with the last of its momentum, climbed up the driver's side door and came to rest directly over the driver's seat.

It had taken an endless, frantic hour to pry the two children out of the wreckage. After that, the rescue squad went to work on the driver's side, but with less urgency; it was obvious to all observers that the driver had not survived. Two members of the rescue squad became physically ill while they worked; all agreed that it was a good thing that the children had been unconscious.

◆ ◆ ◆

The double trauma stat happened to coincide with the afternoon shift change. Nobody goes home during a trauma stat, so there were plenty of people available to work the twin admissions. Mary Fallat circulated back and forth between the two code rooms, but soon ignored Teresa, who was stable, in favor of Tom, who was not. The trauma team rapidly installed all the usual monitors, probes, and intravenous lines, and because Tom's breathing was labored and erratic, the anesthesiologist was forced to intubate him before X-rays had been taken.

Tom's head had been bandaged at the scene, so it was the X-ray that first showed the trauma team how awful the injury really was. The skull was distorted in half a dozen places; it appeared that the entire left side of his head had been crushed. The vertebrae of the neck were stretched apart, and the anesthesiologist winced. She'd had to put in the breathing tube to keep the boy alive, but from the look of that neck, she'd done him no favors. From the sound of the boy's heartbeat, the thought was academic anyway; the *beep-beep-beep* of the monitor had slowed noticeably. One of the symptoms of severe brain damage is bradycardia, a slow heartbeat. Another is falling body temperature. "What's his temp?" the anesthesiologist asked. A nurse reached for a thermometer.

Neurosurgery had been called, of course; the resident had arrived even before the patients. His boss, Dennis Johnson, the attending neurosurgeon, arrived shortly after the resident looked at the X-rays. The attending stared at the X-rays for a long time, and shook his head several times. Then he turned and looked at the boy. The left arm was mangled and bloody, but the uninjured right arm had already twisted, the hand clawlike, facing outward. In the lingo of emergency medicine, this is called posturing. This particular posture simply confirmed what the neurosurgeon already knew: The boy's brain was dying. Finally, he spoke: "If you can stabilize him and get him upstairs, we'll do what we can, but . . ." the sentence hung in the air. There was no need to finish it.

Mary Fallat and the neurosurgeon moved to the other code room, where Teresa's X-rays now also hung on the wall. The neurosurgeon brightened visibly at the sight of the films. "Now there's a manageable injury," he said, pointing out the skull fracture, a dent that would have to be pulled out to relieve pressure on the girl's brain, and the small pool of blood beneath it that would have to be drained. But the skull fracture was comfortably far forward; there would be no damage to the motor and speech areas of the girl's brain. The operation would leave a scar that would show on her forehead, but a good plastic surgeon, or a good hairdresser for that matter, could hide such a scar. The good news was that, absent something unexpected, the girl would recover.

"We'll take the girl first," the neurosurgeon announced, cementing his diagnosis of the boy next door. This is called *triage.* Triage means sorting your patients, tending first to the ones who need help most, and ignoring the ones for whom nothing can be done. Emergency medicine, which has its roots in battlefield medicine, is beyond all else an exercise in realities. One grim reality is that sometimes you have to prioritize.

Minutes later, Tom confirmed the neurosurgeon's analysis by plunging into full cardiac arrest and defying all attempts by the code room team to revive him.

◆ ◆ ◆

A death in the code room is a rare event. If a child has any life at all in him, the code room team can usually fan the spark enough to get him into surgery, following which he dies in the intensive care unit. And sometimes, rarely, a kid who should have died, who everybody agreed was going to die, doesn't. Kids, as Marty Eichelberger constantly reminds his people, are full of surprises. Sometimes there are outright miracles.

A death in the code room makes it tough to believe in miracles. The physicians and nurses who make up the trauma team are not accustomed to defeat, and they do not accept it graciously. Some become angry and snappish; others simply grow remote and aloof and go back to their little corners of the hospital to sulk. The members of the trauma team are people who love kids, and losing somebody else's kid is only slightly less wrenching than losing one of your own.

This holds true for everyone up to and including Dr. Eichelberger, who was there, naturally, standing with Heidi in the hallway outside the code room when Trent Lewis, the social worker, walked up to them. "The father's here," Lewis said. "Do you want to come talk to him?"

Marty grimaced and drew in a long breath. "Yeah, just a minute," he said. He walked to the doorway of code room number two, and caught Mary Fallat's eye. "How soon will you be upstairs?" he asked. The team was preparing to take Teresa to X-ray; the neurosurgeons wanted to see CAT scans before beginning their repair work.

"Five minutes," the chief resident answered. "Maybe less."

"Good. The father's here. I don't want to bring him around here," he said, nodding his head toward the other code room, where a nurse and a junior resident were removing all the tubes and wires from Tom's body, preparing it for the short trip to the hospital morgue. Mary nodded.

Marty turned and walked the few steps back to where Heidi and Trent were waiting. "Okay, let's go," he said. This was nobody's favorite chore, least of all Marty's, but rank does have its responsibilities.

Daniel J. Franklin wore a gray, pin-stripe, three-piece suit, a luxurious-looking white shirt with French cuffs, and a perfectly matched maroon-and-gray-striped necktie. Heidi tried to sneak a look at his socks, but his pants cuffs covered them. The shoes, however, were expensive-looking black loafers. He stood up as Marty, Heidi, and Trent filed into the tiny room. Trent made the introductions; the man shook hands with both Marty and Heidi. Then there was an awkward silence.

"Mr. Franklin," Marty began, "I'm sorry to have to bring you bad news. Your son Tom died just a few minutes ago. We did everything we could to revive him, but his injuries were just too extensive."

Marty shook his head. "I'm sorry," he repeated. "I'm really sorry." The man nodded and blinked his eyes several times. He said nothing.

"Teresa is in stable condition, but she is unconscious. She had a severe blow to the head, and she'll need some surgery to repair the damage. However, based on what we know so far, our neurosurgeons believe she has an excellent chance of recovery. She's on her way to X-ray now for CAT scans; we'll take you up there in a few minutes."

Mr. Franklin nodded again, opened his mouth, paused, then asked, slowly, "What happened to Tom?"

"He had massive injuries to most of his left side," Marty said. "That included a head injury that he simply could not survive. From the extent of the injury, I would say it's unusual that he lived as long as he did."

"Was he conscious?"

"No." Marty shook his head. "Not possible. He must have lost consciousness instantly."

"What about Teresa?"

"She's been unconscious since the accident," Marty said. "She must have had quite a blow to the head; she has what we call a depressed skull fracture. We can repair that, but she may not regain consciousness for a day or two, maybe longer."

Daniel Franklin sat, nodding his head for a few seconds, his eyes on the floor. When he finally spoke, his voice was firm but soft. "You know my wife—I lost my wife in this accident, too." He looked up, smiled a tight-lipped smile. "You're very kind," he said, looking from face to face. "I appreciate everything you've done. I just—I don't know what to say. An hour ago I was in court, in the middle of a trial. All of a sudden half my family's gone. This is not the sort of thing you expect to ever have to deal with." He shook his head again. "I've got so much to do now," he said slowly, "I don't even know where to begin."

◆ ◆ ◆

In the four days that followed, he made arrangements to bury his wife and son. Except for that, he lived at Children's Hospital.

He slept in the ICU waiting room, showered in the residents' locker room, ate in the hospital cafeteria. His car remained in the same parking spot for so long that the security guards checked to make sure it hadn't been abandoned.

Daniel J. Franklin, it developed, was a partner in one of Washington's better-known law firms. His income ran well into six figures. His clients included billionaires, giant corporations, and foreign governments. Even in the cutthroat Washington legal community, he was an acknowledged superstar.

In the blink of an eye, he had lost his wife and his son. His daughter lay unconscious in the hospital. In an instant all the money, all the power, all the status ceased to matter; there was only grief, searing and unspeakable, and that grief, coupled with a lawyer's need to remain in control, translated into an obsessive attachment to all that was left of his family: his daughter, Teresa. He didn't leave because he couldn't.

The ICU nurses urged him to go home and get a good night's sleep. He demurred. A nurse pressed him; he admitted, softly but matter-of-factly, that he didn't have much desire to spend time in an empty house. And that was that. He continued to sleep in the waiting room, wearing a bright blue jogging suit. In the daytime, he changed into slacks and a golf shirt. He stopped wearing a wristwatch.

He spent most of his waking hours at Teresa's bedside, stroking her hands, talking softly to her. He brought in an enormous briefcase stuffed with children's books, which he read aloud to the girl, one after another. At the suggestion of the nurses, he brought a tape recorder and tried to read stories into it, but he kept lapsing into Dictaphone jargon, adding "period, paragraph" and similar comments. He had to try several times before he got one right.

On Saturday, Teresa had begun to thrash about in the bed. By Saturday evening, the movements were purposeful; she seemed to recognize her father's voice and could follow simple instructions from the nurses.

Sunday she opened her eyes and looked around but didn't speak. She appeared oriented, and dutifully squeezed people's fingers and wiggled her toes on request, but she wouldn't answer questions. Her father sat with her, talking, reading stories to her, and several times he bent over the bed to hug her, awkwardly because of all the tubes and gadgets still in use. He left long enough to fetch several stuffed toys, which he arranged around the foot of the girl's bed.

Late Sunday afternoon, they moved Teresa to IMCU. She was stable, had made substantial recovery from her physical injuries, and no longer needed the high-tech ICU environment. And they needed the ICU bed for little David Myers.

◆ ◆ ◆

On her way to IMCU, Heidi was intercepted by Teresa's father. He seemed to have been waiting for her, yet at the same time he seemed to be in a hurry. He drew her into a tiny office just off the ICU waiting room. The office technically belonged to the Department of Social Work, and Leslie Strauss, the social worker who usually handled the ICU, sometimes used it as an office, but most of the time it was used by parents who needed a brief bit of privacy.

"She's talking," Mr. Franklin said.

"Great," said Heidi. "Sounds like she's making real progress."

"She's asking about her mother and Tommy," he continued. "I don't know what to tell her."

Heidi paused for a long moment before answering. "Tell her the truth," she said. "That's the only choice you have. If you lie to a child, they remember it forever." He said nothing. "If Teresa's asking," Heidi said slowly, "it means she's ready to know."

Letting out a long breath, he said, "Okay. I guess there's no such thing as a good time. This won't . . . hurt her chances of recovery, will it?"

Heidi shook her head. "She's making very good progress. She'll be sad, of course; she'll go through a grieving process, just like you are. It's a natural process. You shouldn't try to stop it, or avoid it." She stood up. "Would you like me to go with you?"

Mr. Franklin stood up slowly. He looked profoundly unhappy, but when he spoke, his voice was even and firm. "Yes," he said. "Yes, I'd appreciate it very much."

◆ ◆ ◆

Aside from the head wound, Teresa's only other injury was a broken left forearm. It might have gone unnoticed, but the trauma team routinely performs a head-to-toe exam on unconscious children. An orthopedic resident set the arm while the plastic surgeon was working his magic on Teresa's scalp wound. The fracture would heal cleanly; the arm would be fine in a matter of weeks.

The neurosurgeons had carefully opened the scalp around the skull fracture and, working with delicate precision, had put everything back in place. There was, of course, some damage to the brain itself, but as evidenced by Teresa's rapid return to consciousness, the damage was not permanent. She appeared to have a full range of motion and sensation, her vision was unimpaired, her hearing intact, and when she spoke, her words—though blurry—were understandable.

The surgeons had had to cut away some of her chestnut brown hair in order to do their repair work, and now a neat bandage covered the left side of her head, from her forehead back almost to her ear. The lone remaining IV line was taped to the back of her right hand. She lay in bed, propped up on two pillows, surrounded by stuffed animals and storybooks. Her eyes were focused and alert.

"Hi, Teresa," Heidi began. "My name's Heidi. You don't remember, but I was here when you came into the hospital. I found this guy," she pointed a thumb at Teresa's father, "out in the hallway. He says he knows you. Should I trust him?"

Teresa giggled. "That's my daddy," she said.

"So how are you feeling?" Heidi asked. "Are you feeling okay? You look a whole lot better." The girl nodded her head, but said nothing. Heidi looked across the bed at Teresa's father. He opened his mouth, started to speak, cleared his throat, then tried again.

"Honey, I have to tell you some bad news," he said. Heidi could hear the voice begin to waver. She glanced up; the man's face was turning red, his eyes were starting to fill with tears. Mr. Franklin turned his face away; his daughter looked at him, then at Heidi.

"Teresa," Heidi began, "you know you were hurt in a car wreck, and now you're getting better." It was a statement, not a question. Teresa nodded.

"You know that your mom and your brother were hurt in the car wreck, too, don't you?" Another nod.

"Well, they were hurt a whole lot worse than you were. You're going to be okay, but they were hurt so bad that they couldn't get better, and they both died. We're all very sad about that." She stopped, waited. No commentary, no philosophizing, just the facts. If Teresa wanted to know more, she would ask.

She didn't. Teresa looked at Heidi for a long moment, then turned her head so she could look at her father. He was sitting in an armchair on the other side of the bed, his eyes shut, tears streaming down his face, his body shaking. Teresa stared at him for a long moment, then looked back at Heidi. Her eyes were beginning to fill with tears.

"Sometimes daddies cry, too, Teresa," Heidi said softly. "It's okay to cry; that's what people do when they're sad."

Teresa closed her eyes. Tears rolled down the sides of her face. She began to sob.

Heidi stood, saying nothing, for several seconds. Then she left, closing the door quietly behind her.

Eleven

When Herta Feely came to Children's Hospital as a public-relations consultant for the trauma program, she would have been the first to describe herself as a seasoned PR person, hard-eyed and cynical. She had at various times worked for newspapers, wire services, magazines, television stations; she had paid plenty of dues. She knew the territory; during ten years in the communications business, she had done it all, from publicity work for Amnesty International to pushing oil products for Chevron. Then she had moved to Washington, and into every PR person's ambition—successful free-lance work.

Washington is a public relations dream town, where every business or organization needs a publicist, a media adviser, an ad agency, or all three. Communications, getting the word out to the faithful, is the lifeblood of the political process, and in the nation's capital it has been refined into an art form. There are only a few cities in the world where a good PR person can earn as much as a good lawyer; Washington, D.C., is one of them.

That, ultimately, is what attracted Herta from California. The West Coast was a wonderful place, vibrant and full of opportunity, but also full of noble causes—a weakness of Herta's. She had to resist the urge to pursue them; noble causes were soul-satisfying but did little for the checking account. Corporate public relations paid well, but Herta chafed at the white-collar sweatshop environment. Free-lance work, with no bosses to give orders or share the profits, was best. After a few years at a large Washington PR firm, Herta set out on her own. She edited a newsletter for the World Bank; she served as spokesperson for a national organization and did occasional publicist work for a couple of friendly ad agencies.

Publicist is the modern word for *press agent.* A publicist's job is to get media exposure for a client, thus obtaining for free the public awareness that would otherwise have to be generated by paid advertising. A publicist's clients may range from activists with causes to proclaim to politicians with polls to influence, singers with new records to sell, actors with new movies to tout, or authors with new books to promote. Every client has something to peddle; it is the publicist's challenge to package that something well enough to attract the interest of news reporters, feature writers, or best of all, producers of radio and television talk shows.

Talk shows and publicists coexist in a symbiotic relationship. Without publicists to feed them ideas, most talk shows would go bust. Talk show producers are always hungry for material, and a publicist who speaks the language of broadcasting, and who understands the needs of the producers, can usually get talk show exposure for any client capable of forming complete sentences.

When, in 1985, an ad agency called Herta to inquire if she'd like to do some publicity for a film about Children's Hospital, her reaction was immediate interest mixed with a little apprehension. Doing publicity for a hospital usually meant trying to get doctors on the air, and that was an enterprise fraught with peril. Doctors often did very poorly on television. Nervous physicians hide inside clouds of medical jargon, and that makes for an excruciatingly bad interview. A really bad doc could wreck a whole talk show segment. Two or three really bad ones could wreck a publicist's reputation with talk show producers. On the other hand, a really good doc, someone who could simplify complex medical concepts and express them in English, could do wonders. Herta said she'd meet with them and see what she could do.

The doc she put on television, of course, was Marty Eichelberger, and the film was *Our Children's War,* a fast-paced documentary about the Children's Hospital trauma program. She couldn't have asked for a better setup: The movie was riveting; Eichelberger was charming, handsome, articulate, and perfectly at ease on television. More important, he had something to talk about: the need for children's trauma centers. Most important of all, there were lots of little children whose lives had been saved by Dr. Eichelberger's trauma service, who had grateful parents, and who looked absolutely enchanting on television. Herta spread Eichelberger and his miracle kids all over Washington, and got him on talk shows in six other cities where the documentary was being shown. The exposure generated additional local publicity, and the trauma service received numerous inquiries from physicians in several cities who were interested in starting pediatric trauma services in their own hospitals.

The stated purpose of the DeVore Trust grant had been to offer training in pediatric trauma care. As it had turned out, the first step in the training process was convincing the public and the medical community that there was a need for it. Films like *Our Children's War* were part of that drive. So was publicity, Marty realized, after he got back from his promotional tour and started returning all the phone calls that had come in. Afterward, he phoned Herta. Would she be interested in doing more of the same for the trauma program?

There was no question. Herta was already hooked. She'd been hooked from the moment she had watched the film she had been hired to promote. Here was a cause above all others: saving the lives of little children. Herta, like many professional women, had put off having children, but the craving was there and she adored kids. She had been awed, sometimes almost overwhelmed, as she had roamed the hallways at Children's Hospital; all the kids were so cute, so lovable. And clearly, everyone on the staff loved kids. The office where Herta had a desk was just beyond the nursing station on the fourth floor surgical wing; every time she walked past the nursing station, there were kids all around, some sitting in tiny chairs, some with IVs in their arms, some crawling on the bright blue carpeting. The nurses, who never dressed like nurses, often sat right on the floor with the kids, keeping the toddlers company even while they worked on their endless paperwork.

She knew from watching the film that Marty had designed a new approach to treating injured kids, an approach that was apparently much, much better than what was available to most kids in the country. And Marty was asking her to help spread the word. Now *that* was a noble cause. Yes, she told Marty. Hell, yes.

For more than a year, Herta continued to do publicity work for the hospital on a consulting basis. She stood outside the code room, toured the ICU, sat on the floor and played with the kids outside the 4-Blue nursing station. She fielded questions from local news organizations, arranged interviews for Marty, and occasionally booked Marty or other staff members for speaking engagements. And always she looked for ways to spread the word.

There were two natural advantages to the job: For one thing, this was a hospital in the nation's capital, the second home of all the major news organizations. A producer at NBC once called Herta for advice on rehabilitation centers for children; they wanted to do a segment for the "Today" show. During the conversation, Herta invited the producer to come visit Children's Hospital and see what goes on before the trip to the rehab center. Once the producer got inside the building, of course, she, too, became enchanted with the cute kids who crawl around outside 4-Blue. When the segment ran on the "Today" show, it was all about Children's Hospital and not about rehab centers.

But Herta's biggest inspiration came during one of her late-afternoon chats with Marty. One of Marty's favorite verbal rampages is about accidents. Most of them, he insists, are preventable, and it is the grownups, he insists, who are responsible. Marty is always gentle with parents (another of his favorite speeches is how the injured child also has an injured family). But privately, the stress of seeing so many kids hurt because someone didn't buckle a seat belt, or didn't put away the power tools, or because someone wasn't watching the kid as they should, or the light sockets weren't covered, or the Drano was left out, or the iron was left plugged in, or the window was left open, or kids were playing in the street because there were no playgrounds, or the landlord had never installed smoke detectors, or a hundred other things—eventually it makes a man angry, and Marty was no exception. When the door was safely closed, Marty would proclaim fiercely that there are no accidents. It was an extreme view, mostly a way for Marty to blow off steam, but he spoke with conviction. There are no accidents; there are only acts of negligence. *Accident* is a word we use to excuse our own failure, to ease our own guilt.

About the sixth time Herta heard the speech, she interrupted. "So why aren't we doing something about it?"

Marty stopped in midsentence. "What would you suggest?"

The idea tumbled out in a rush. Why not, Herta said, have a national campaign on accident prevention? Pull out all the stops—make public service announcements on television and radio, form community organizations, get the president to proclaim Child Safety Week. . . .

"The president?" Marty asked.

"How can he refuse?" Herta said. "Nancy Reagan comes here every Christmas and gives toys to the kids. It's for the kids, Marty, injured kids. People'll do anything to help kids. They might even practice accident prevention if we can show them there's a problem."

Marty thought about it for a moment. "Can we raise the money to do it?"

"If we can't, then we won't do it," Herta said.

"Okay, do it. Do it big. See if you can put all of us out of jobs."

Twelve _____

The burn unit at Children's Hospital is on the third floor, a corridor away from the intensive care unit. The ICU is in the Blue section of the hospital, the burn unit in Green. The two units share a common waiting room, a large room full of chairs and couches, just outside the ICU doors.

Inside the burn unit Richard, the four-year-old with the oddly symmetrical burns on his forearms, slept soundly in a bed that was probably far more comfortable and safer than the one he was accustomed to. The nurses are always especially kind to kids like Richard; as soon as he got to the burn unit they got the rest of his clothes off him, bathed him, washed his hair, dressed him in the yellow circus-print pajamas that are standard issue at Children's, and chatted and cooed with him until he finally began to smile and even to talk a little.

They also discovered his great weakness: ice cream. They'd had a tough time in the beginning when they tried to bathe him; he seemed strangely afraid of baths. When he realized he had no choice, he froze up and became stoic, but he relaxed when the nurses let him choose the water temperature he wanted.

His arms were still red, but with the soothing ointment, he seemed comfortable enough and, after the bath, when the nurses had offered him ice cream, he let the nurses feed him the first spoonful, then took over and fed himself the rest. Then, when he was finished, he began crying for no apparent reason. It was the first time he'd cried since coming to the hospital. The nurses, who understand such things, cuddled him and let him cry awhile, then gave him more ice cream.

One of the surgical residents stopped by; he did a cursory examination of Richard and nodded knowingly when the nurses described how differently the boy behaved in the presence of adult males. He had begun to loosen up, and accept hugs from the nurses, and even to talk a bit, but when the resident walked in, the boy had stiffened, and while he had been perfectly polite and responsive, he was clearly tense and answered the resident's questions in monosyllables.

"I'm not surprised," the resident told the nurses. "I saw his X-rays." Whenever the trauma staff suspects that a child has been the victim of abuse, they often order a whole-body X-ray. Although the official memorandum interpreting the X-rays would not be put into Richard's medical record for several hours yet, the news travels faster. "Evidence of at least two and maybe three old fractures," the resident said grimly, "all of which appear to have healed on their own. Somebody has really banged this kid around."

The nurses shook their heads. How could anybody deliberately hurt such a cute kid? Finally one of the nurses spoke up, to no one in particular. "You think it would hurt to give him a little more ice cream?"

◆ ◆ ◆

Down the hallway, outside the closed double doors that isolate the burn unit from the rest of the floor, Richard's mother spent the night in the ICU waiting room, where her disheveled appearance fit right in with the other haggard-looking parents who slept there. Twice during the night she roused and phoned the nurses in the burn unit. "He's fine. He has a fever, but he's resting comfortably, and he's doing fine," the nurses reassured the mother. The part about the fever was true; Richard had a temperature of ninety-nine, which was not at all alarming, but was a good excuse to keep Richard under wraps. The nurses did not invite the mother to visit.

When the mother called the third time, the nurses let her come see Richard, but first they tacked elaborate Isolation and Infection Hazard signs on the door to Richard's room, and they dressed the mother in a sterile gown and cap before escorting her into the room. Richard seemed genuinely glad to see her, hugged her gingerly, and cried a little at first, but then he insisted on hugging the two nurses who were in the room with them. "I got ice cream," he told his mother solemnly.

After a few minutes the nurses declared visiting hours over, and the mother dutifully went back to the waiting room. The nurses caucused, and after several minutes' discussion concluded that the mother might not be the primary culprit. The boy's reactions had been, for him, appropriate. They made extensive notations in Richard's medical record and had a long chat with the nurses who relieved them at shift change.

Shortly after shift change, a physician from the Division of Child Protection came to the burn unit, examined Richard, and read the notes in Richard's medical record. The nurses mentioned the X-rays, and the physician phoned the radiology department for details. Then she phoned the Washington, D.C., Department of Human Services, and after that, the police.

An hour later, the physician, a D.H.S. social worker, and a police detective met with Richard's mother and her fiancé, who had arrived at the ICU waiting room only a few minutes earlier. The confrontation was low-key, almost gentle, but businesslike.

"Our concern," the physician explained, "is for Richard's welfare. That's the most important thing. I think we all agree on that." The couple nodded.

"We are especially troubled because Richard's injuries don't match the explanation we've gotten about how those injuries occurred. This has caused us to be concerned that Richard has been a victim of child abuse.

"Whenever we think there's a possibility of child abuse, the law requires us to notify the appropriate authorities and take steps to protect the child, and we have done that. Richard is safe, I can assure you, and is receiving excellent care. The next step is to try to piece together exactly what did happen to Richard yesterday, and we hope you'll work with us and help us. I know that you want what's best for Richard, just as we do."

Child abuse, the physician knew from long experience, doesn't happen in a vacuum. It almost never happens in cold blood, only in anger. Figure out the underlying circumstances, and you can often fix the problem. Establishing some kind of communication with the parents is the first step in that process.

But meanwhile, until everything could be sorted out, the physician explained, the state had assumed temporary custody of Richard and had gotten a court order requiring someone from the hospital to accompany Richard's mother, or her fiancé, whenever they visited Richard.

Throughout the conversation, Richard's mother nodded quietly. At one point, she brushed away a tear. Her fiancé remained polite but grew visibly more tense as the conversation progressed. Finally, he stood up, excused himself, and walked out of the room. He did not return.

Thirteen

Dr. Riad Karmy-Jones learned about David Myers when he reported to work at 5:00 A.M. Surgical residents get a day off every other weekend and usually spend the day sleeping. Karmy-Jones, who appeared not to require sleep, had spent the day sightseeing in Washington.

Officially, Karmy-Jones was at Children's to study general pediatric surgery for three months, and, indeed, he had watched, and had often assisted in, major and minor surgery of almost every kind. But what attracted him most were the trauma cases. He intended to make trauma his surgical specialty. In his native Canada, trauma medicine was still largely an ad hoc matter, left to individual hospitals. Some were very good, others very bad. The Canadian Parliament had recently been acting to change that, and before long trauma care would be an official part of Canada's National Health System. Karmy-Jones would be one of the first U.S.–trained traumatologists to work in that new system.

It was K-J's habit to make a quick tour of the ICU the first item on his morning agenda; any overnight trauma cases, any interesting ones, would be there. This particular morning he spotted little David as soon as he rounded the corner, buttonholed David's nurse for five minutes of details, then headed for the nursing station to read David's chart. By the time everyone mustered for rounds at six, K-J knew as much about David's case as anyone in the hospital.

Bedside rounds are a firm tradition at every teaching hospital. They ensure that every resident knows the daily progress of every case on his service so that, somewhere in his career when he sees another case just like it, he will at least have a reference point. The advantage to the patient is a great deal of attention from a great many doctors. Residents are M.D.'s doing postgraduate work in their chosen specialty. Surgical residencies last four or five years, following which the

100

surgeon is eligible to begin working toward final and formal certification by the American Board of Surgery. Meanwhile, the operative word is *work*. Residents provide cheap skilled labor at teaching hospitals, and in most teaching hospitals they work brutal hours.

Children's is no exception. Residents are on call one day out of three. The day they are on call, they must stay all night in the hospital, where they are available to the nursing staff for any questions or problems that may arise. If there are no problems, the residents can sleep, but there are few nights when there are no problems. At 6:00 A.M., the resident goes off call but does not go home. The off-call day is a normal work day—beginning with bedside rounds at 6:00 A.M., followed by a full day in the OR, observing or assisting one of the five staff surgeons, and ending with evening bedside rounds which begin whenever the OR schedule is complete. Residents are grateful when the work day lasts only twelve hours.

There are two surgical chief residents at Children's. A chief resident is a finished surgeon who desires additional intensive training in pediatric surgery. Chief residents are hired for overlapping two-year terms, called fellowships. The chief residents supervise all the other residents, deciding which residents will assist or observe which operations, who will work what schedule, and so on. Chief residents also decide what time morning rounds will be held.

Mary Fallat, the senior chief resident, liked to start at 6:00 A.M., which usually meant the rest of the residents had to get there at 5:00 A.M. to check on all their cases. Residents quickly learned that it was unwise in the extreme to be unprepared when Mary Fallat conducted rounds. Fallat—gentle, soft-spoken, and unfailingly polite—had an almost supernatural ability to ask the one question a resident was not prepared to answer. Residents had been known to pull out their old medical textbooks to bone up before rounds; Fallat appeared to remember every word of every textbook she'd ever read, and she had a stubborn notion that bedside rounds should be used for teaching such things to the residents.

Rounds begin in the intensive care nursery, an almost surrealistic place where tiny infants lie unmoving in bassinets, swathed in tubing and dwarfed by the gleaming machinery that keeps them alive. A small but predictable percentage of all children are born with birth defects; of that number, an equally predictable majority can be made whole by surgery. Children's Hospital attracts patients from all over the world, and many of them are attracted by the reputation of Dr. Judson Randolph, who has made the surgical repair of birth defects his personal specialty. At any given time, the intensive care nursery will have two dozen or more recovering infants.

Most of Mary Fallat's residents will go on to be general surgeons and will never personally attempt any of the highly sophisticated and delicate operations, such as transforming a hermaphrodite into a little girl, or even the very mundane procedures, such as removing a sixth finger or toe. But having seen many such cases, they will remember in a general way what was done and what the outcome was, and they will know how to counsel distraught parents and where to send such patients for treatment.

The residents, some in scrub suits, some in street clothes, all with sterile gowns draped around them, clustered around the first bassinet. It is necessary to stand close during ICN rounds; voices must be kept soft.

"Who has this patient?" Fallat asked. A resident straightened, cleared his throat. Fallat nodded, and the resident launched into the standard presentation.

"Barbara is six weeks old, and this is her third postop day following an NEC resection," the resident intoned.

There are always NEC babies in the intensive care nursery; NEC is short for *necrotizing enterocolitis,* an inflammation of the bowel so severe that, left untreated, it destroys the bowel and kills the infant. The standard surgical therapy is to open the abdomen, snip off the inflamed portion of intestine, then close the incision partway, leaving the two cut ends of the intestine in view so that the surgeons can make sure the inflammation will not return. Once they are sure, they can suture the bowel back together, and the child can go home.

"Barbara's vital signs are all stable," the resident droned on, reciting heart rate, blood pressure, temperature, and other relevant numbers. "She appears to be progressing normally and without complication."

"When would you close the ileostomy?" Fallat asked.

The resident stopped with his mouth open. He knew that the cut ends of the bowel were kept outside the child's abdomen so that the child would not become infected by his own waste. He also knew that at least once every day he had to inspect the ileostomy, looking for signs of inflammation. And he knew that the nurses kept close watch over the baby's temperature, and that she had been free of fever for several days. But when to repair the bowel? . . . The question hung in the air.

Fallat tried again. "At what point will it be appropriate to repair the bowel and close the incision?"

The resident answered slowly, carefully. "I would say that when we are satisfied that the inflammation will not recur, it would be appropriate to close the incision."

Fallat nodded. "Right. And how will we know that?" This time the resident was stumped. Fallat let the question hang a few seconds, then answered it herself. "When Barbara begins to thrive, we will know that her intestine has begun to function again. So when she begins to grow, to gain weight, assuming she has remained afebrile, then that is the appropriate time to consider closing the ileostomy." She turned away, and the crowd of residents moved a few feet and reclustered around the next bassinet. "Who has this child?" Fallat asked.

◆ ◆ ◆

It was close to 7:00 A.M. by the time Fallat and the clump of surgical residents reached the bedside of little David Myers. Fallat smiled when Karmy-Jones spoke up unprompted and began reciting David's story as though he had personally admitted him.

"David's a four-point-five-year-old male struck by a car and thrown fifty feet. He has a closed head injury, bilateral pulmonary contusions, bilateral femur fractures. And a broken clavicle," he added, to be complete. Nobody cared about the clavicle.

"He has not been conscious since the accident," Karmy-Jones went on, "and he has become progressively less stable over the last several hours."

The dilemma, Karmy-Jones explained, was that David's injuries tended to feed on themselves and grow. His head injury had caused his blood pressure to drop, while causing the pressure inside his skull to go up. If the pressure inside the skull exceeded the pressure inside the arteries, then no blood would circulate to the brain and the patient would die. Already, overnight, David had had several crises when blood pressure had dropped and cranial pressure had risen to within a few perilous points of each other. In one case, the ICU physicians had had to open the pressure monitor in David's skull and simply let the excess fluid drain out. After that, they gave David diuretics to flush out excess fluids and kept his blood pressure artificially elevated by injecting Adrenalin into his intravenous lines.

Karmy-Jones took a deep breath. He still wasn't finished. Matters were made worse, he said, by David's lung injuries. The bruises on his lungs made it necessary to keep David's respirator operating with positive end expiratory pressure; unfortunately, PEEP also causes cranial pressure to rise, and therein lay the true dilemma: The treatment for the injury might be as fatal as the injury itself.

The ICU physicians had carefully straddled the fence all night, keeping the respirator at the minimum setting capable of producing good blood gas readings and fighting the bouts of increased cranial pressure as they came, one by one. So far they had been successful, and David appeared to be stabilizing at this time, but the boy was still on very shaky ground.

"The next twenty-four to forty-eight hours are critical," Karmy-Jones observed. "If we can keep him relatively stable for that period, then he has a good chance of recovering to some degree." It was a grim assessment: to some degree. Translated, it meant David might very well die. Or he might survive to be a vegetable. Or he might only be seriously crippled. It was a poor set of choices.

Over the next two days, Karmy-Jones all but adopted little David Myers. He visited the bedside almost hourly, chatted with Mr. and Mrs. Myers, answered their questions, even took them to the X-ray department to show them David's CAT scans and explain the significance of the brain swelling. Several times a day, he tracked down Mary Fallat for consultations. This was not merely etiquette; residents do not make medical decisions without first getting the chief resident's approval. Mary Fallat, in turn, consults with Marty Eichelberger several times a day. Through this chain of command, Dr. Eichelberger personally—albeit indirectly—supervises the treatment of every child admitted to the trauma service. But even though Drs. Eichelberger and Fallat were directing David's care, it was Karmy-Jones who applied it.

At the bedside, K-J was forever fine-tuning the treatment, adjusting the mix of oxygen and air flowing through David's respirator, adding this drug or that one, discontinuing some other. Gradually, David grew more and more stable. The fluctuations in blood pressure grew less, and when K-J experimentally stopped giving David Adrenalin, the blood pressure dropped a little but then stayed steady. The cranial pressure monitor showed a figure that varied less and less, staying safely in the high teens.

At Tuesday morning rounds, K-J suggested that it was time to discontinue the drug that was keeping David paralyzed. As long as he remained paralyzed, K-J argued, it was impossible to wean him off the respirator, and indeed it was impossible even to tell if he was ready to begin the weaning process. This should be done quickly, he argued; patients left too long on a respirator become physically dependent on it; the longer they stay hooked up to the machine, the harder it is to wean them away from it. There was general agreement among the surgical residents and, more important, the chief resident agreed. By midmorning, the last dose of Pavulon had worn off, and David responded by swinging his legs, and occasionally moving one arm. He did not open his eyes.

By the time rounds were conducted on Wednesday, David's eyelids had begun to flutter, and he had begun to assist in his own breathing. K-J had gradually reduced the setting of the respirator, and David was making up the difference. The breaths were shallow, but they were there, and the computerized display at the bedside showed a respiration count in the forties and fifties, as David's lungs matched the mechanical efforts of the respirator. If he continues to progress, K-J said, we should try to extubate him tomorrow. Everyone agreed.

◆ ◆ ◆

The nurses in the ICU routinely shoo parents out and into the waiting room just before the residents arrive for morning rounds. Part of that is tradition, a tradition that says you always keep the number of people in the ICU to a minimum. Another part is precaution: Residents on rounds tend to speak bluntly and to speculate, sometimes inaccurately, about a patient's condition and prognosis. There are discussions, and sometimes disagreements, about which way to proceed. Such discussions are entirely proper in a teaching environment, and the bedside gathering is, if nothing else, a classroom with legs. Ultimately, the patients benefit from the dozen-odd second opinions.

But parents, the ICU nurses have learned, do not. They often resent listening while their child is discussed abstractly; more important, they often know just enough medical lingo to understand some of the more pessimistic comments. To make matters even worse, the residents on rounds are always in a hurry. They have several dozen cases to discuss each morning, so they move from bed to bed rapidly, spending little if any time on explanations or courtesies. So if a parent happens to be in earshot and has become alarmed at what he overhears, he will certainly become angry as well when the group of doctors abruptly leaves without offering explanations or reassurances.

The ICU nurses long ago decided that parents did not need or deserve such aggravation, so the firm rule is that parents have to leave during rounds.

David and Patricia Myers didn't particularly mind when it was time to move to the waiting room; at 6:00 A.M., whoever was at little David's bedside was usually exhausted, and grateful for a chance to sink into one of the soft couches in the ICU waiting room. It was one of the few predictable, routine events in their lives at the moment.

On Sunday, the shock and grief had been a private matter just for Mr. and Mrs. Myers. By Sunday night, Pat's mother and younger brother had arrived from Georgia, and the four of them slept—or tried to sleep—in the waiting room. This was highly unsatisfactory since there was only limited couch space available, so they began shuttling back and forth between the hospital and the Myers's apartment.

Then on Monday, the visits and the phone calls began. Cards arrived from friends and acquaintances at the FBI, at the weather service, at their church. Pat's fellow secretaries in the FBI's public affairs office took up a collection and bought a stuffed animal for little David. It was delivered, in person, by Pat's boss, a deputy director of the FBI.

The phone at the apartment rang constantly, and before long so did the phone in the ICU waiting room, as more people learned that number. David and Patricia Myers had not thought of themselves as socializing people; they were impressed, sometimes almost overwhelmed, at the outpouring of sympathy and support from friends, relatives, coworkers.

After the chaos of the first few days, they settled into a sort of routine. One of them always stayed at the hospital; one of them was always there, around the clock; the other would take the car and run errands, go shopping, tend to the everyday chores. Pat's mother took charge of the apartment and made sure everything stayed in order there; her brother learned the route between the apartment and the hospital, so he could help with the chauffeuring duties.

Most important, they divided up bedside duty. Most of the time, David and Pat themselves stayed with little David. One would sleep while the other sat at the bedside. After a few hours, they would switch places. Except when the nurses shooed them out during rounds, one or the other of them was nearly always in the ICU.

Pat was there when the child in the adjacent bed died. There is scant privacy to be gained from the thin curtains that can be drawn around an ICU bed; Pat, sitting close to little David's bed and squeezing his hand, heard every word, every shriek and sob from the parents, until one of the ICU nurses, with a briskness that surprised and angered Pat, ordered her to wait outside. Pat's own nerves were frayed by worry and lack of sleep; once in the waiting room she sat, seething, for a long time. Then she cried for awhile. Finally, she fell asleep.

◆ ◆ ◆

Shortly before 9:00 A.M. on Thursday morning, Karmy-Jones assembled a small team of physicians and nurses at little David's bedside. Mary Fallat had approved the decision at rounds that morning, but now, with an anesthesiologist, a neurosurgery resident, and a specialist from the ICU all present, K-J went over the facts one more time.

"We've weaned him down to minimal settings," he said, nodding at the respirator. "His cranial pressure has been steady for the last two days, and despite the fact that he has not fully regained consciousness, he appears to be ready to breathe on his own. Can anyone think of any reason not to extubate him?"

The doctors exchanged glances and shrugs. One by one, they looked at K-J and shook their heads. No objection, doctor. Proceed.

With a final glance at the monitors, K-J began peeling away the mask of adhesive tape that held the respirator tube firmly in place. Little David's eyelids fluttered slightly as the tape came away, leaving tiny white flecks of adhesive clinging to his skin.

When the tube was completely free, K-J grasped the blue plastic tube that led to the respirator. He looked at the bank of electronic monitors once more; pulse was 110, respiration 44, cranial pressure 10. He looked at the anesthesiologist; the anesthesiologist nodded and stepped forward. As K-J stepped back, he popped the respirator hose off the airway tube.

The respirator alarm filled the ICU with a high-pitched peeping noise. David's ICU nurse edged around the group, adjusted the controls on the respirator, and the peeping was replaced by a tense silence.

The anesthesiologist placed his left hand over David's jaw, grasping the airway tube with his right. With one swift, continuous motion he drew the tube out of David's windpipe. White mucus dripped from the plastic tube; the anesthesiologist tossed it into a trash can. No one spoke. All eyes were on little David's chest. It didn't move.

The instinct to breathe is the most primitive of all instincts, yet it is based on a complex interaction of brain cells, nerve cells, and blood chemistry. As the cells of the body use oxygen from the bloodstream, they replace it with carbon dioxide. Sensor nerves measure the carbon dioxide level in the blood, and as it increases, the nerves send increasingly strong signals to a tiny area near the base of the brain that, in turn, sends increasingly urgent messages to the diaphragm. Eventually, the diaphragm flexes, expanding the lungs and bringing a fresh supply of oxygen into the body.

The sweep second hand on the wall clock moved a quarter circle, then a half. It took forty seconds for little David to take his first spontaneous breath, a loud, rasping gasp that filled his lungs to capacity. Five seconds later, he took a second breath, then a third, then a fourth. The breaths were labored and jerky, but they were breaths. The team at David's bedside began to relax.

Then the neurosurgeon, his face impassive, pointed a finger at the bank of monitors. The pressure inside David's head had begun to increase. As K-J watched, it climbed past 20, 21, 22, 25. . . .

"Come on, David, just relax and breathe for us," K-J said aloud. As he spoke, he reached over and stroked David's forehead. "Breathe for us, David."

David's chest heaved erratically, several shallow breaths followed by deep gasping ones, followed by long pauses. The intracranial pressure monitor continued to climb, 38 . . . 40 . . . 44. . . .

"What's the limit?" K-J asked the neurosurgery resident.

"He can tolerate it for a while," the neuro man replied. "Let's see where it peaks."

David's breathing became more rhythmic, but also more rapid. The anesthesiologist held a hissing oxygen mask near David's mouth and nose. The extra oxygen seemed to help a little; the rasping breaths became quieter, but still rapid and shallow, almost panting. The entire team stood, saying nothing, all eyes fixed on the cranial pressure monitor. The number was climbing more slowly now, but as the team watched, it jumped from 50 to 52, then 54 . . . 55 . . . 58. . . .

"How much?" K-J again asked.

"Not yet, not yet. Wait for a peak," the neurosurgery resident answered.

David's breaths were rapid and shallow. Just below the cranial pressure figure on the electronic readout, a second number showed David's respiration rate: It was steady at 70, more than one breath a second. The cranial pressure monitor read 64.

"Any theories?" K-J asked the neurosurgeon.

"Whatever it is, he's not ventilating right," the neuro man answered. "Maybe it's the lung contusion. Maybe he has some sort of mild airway obstruction. Maybe that part of his brain is damaged. All I can tell you for certain is that he's not behaving the way I would like him to." As he spoke, the cranial pressure reading passed 70, then 71 . . . 74 . . . 77. "Okay, we're getting into the danger zone now," the neurosurgeon said.

K-J looked at the anesthesiologist, who nodded. There was no need for discussion. The anesthesiologist pressed the oxygen mask firmly over David's mouth and nose and began rhythmically squeezing the black bag attached to the mask, forcing pure oxygen into David's lungs. The cranial pressure reading reached 84, then began to move downward, 82 . . . 78 . . . 75. . . .

"Pretty clearly a respiratory problem," K-J observed to his neurosurgeon colleague.

"Not necessarily," the neurosurgeon replied. "You could get the same result from a brain lesion. I'm going to order another CAT scan; if this is the result of brain swelling, then we can hope it will get better as the swelling decreases. If the swelling is gone, then we have to consider the possibility that the damage is permanent."

K-J stared bleakly at the tiny body on the bed. As he watched, the anesthesiologist expertly slipped a fresh airway tube into David's windpipe, taped it securely into place, and reattached David to the respirator. The cranial pressure was down to 43 . . . 41 . . . 40. Nursing homes are full of ventilator-dependent, brain-damaged patients; it is a phenomenon created by the advent of trauma centers. Before the days of the Children's Hospital Trauma Center, little David would surely have died of his injuries; with sophisticated machinery, experienced physicians, and expert nursing care, the trauma team had kept him alive. Each day his chances of survival had improved, and now he was almost certain to live. But for what?

As he turned and walked away from the bedside, Karmy-Jones wondered, for the first time, whether they had done little David any favors.

Fourteen _____

In most hospitals it would be unusual to see rehabilitation notes in the medical record of an unconscious patient. But Children's is no ordinary hospital, and Cyndy Wright is no ordinary rehab nurse.

The marriage of trauma care with rehabilitation is a natural one, but historically it has been awkward and sometimes fractious. Rehabilitation, like anesthesiology, has had a long-standing, and undeserved, reputation as one of medicine's backwaters.

The surgeons who became traumatologists realized two decades ago that anesthesiologists had to be part of the trauma team; anesthesiologists are trained to provide artificial life support, to breathe for patients, control their heartbeat and circulation with drugs, and keep them alive while their injuries—which would once have been fatal—can be repaired. With anesthesiologists on trauma teams, the survival rates went up dramatically.

And in equally dramatic numbers, the trauma centers began producing cripples. People who once would have died of their injuries now survived, but often they survived with severe, lingering injuries. A significant portion of trauma patients left the trauma centers and went into nursing homes; a few went to rehabilitation centers. Over time, some of them improved. Others wasted away and finally died.

It took years for traumatologists to realize that trauma rehabilitation was exactly like trauma resuscitation: The earlier you started it, the better the results. Now many of the major trauma centers have rehabilitation divisions, whose job it is to begin planning a course of restorative therapy almost as soon as the patient comes into the hospital.

The Children's Trauma Service has Cyndy Wright.

When medical people say the word *rehab,* they often give it a little extra twist, the sort of inflection you might hear if they had said "pain in the ass," instead. Two decades ago, the same inflection was often

111

applied to the words *trauma* and *traumatologist.* Today, it is the rehab people who are fighting to elevate their specialty to something beyond mere aftercare. It is still a new idea, and medicine is always slow to change its ways; it is only natural, then, that rehab people have acquired a reputation for treading on toes, interfering in the business of other specialties, picking arguments, and, worst of all, winning them.

Cyndy is ideally suited to the profession; she comes from a long line of instigators and agitators. Forty years ago, her grandmother defied the rules at the Oregon State College for the Deaf and taught the students sign language as well as lipreading. A dozen years ago her father, while chief librarian at Gallaudet College, shut down the entire library and refused to reopen it until the college added wheelchair ramps. Cyndy herself has childhood memories of being with her mother and father in civil rights marches back in the early sixties, long before civil rights was a popular cause.

Cyndy is the third generation in her family to work around people with disabilities; she started doing volunteer work with autistic children while still in high school. She worked easily with children, and that, too, was no accident: Her mother, a college professor, was an expert in child development and education, specializing in preschoolers. By the time she was a teenager, Cyndy knew more about small kids than many mothers do. After she finished nursing school, she joined the staff at Children's Hospital to work with kids who had congenital disabilities—things like Down's syndrome, cerebral palsy, brittle bone disease. The work was emotionally draining but ultimately satisfying; it was always possible to make life a little better for disabled kids, if you knew how to handle them.

Cyndy arrived at Children's Hospital just about the same time that Marty Eichelberger did, and as his trauma service grew increasingly sophisticated, Cyndy began to notice. One day she stopped him in a hallway and pointed an accusing finger at him. "As if we didn't have enough to do with all the disabled kids who were born that way," she said with mock seriousness, "now you've created a whole new class of disabilities with your trauma service. What are you going to do about it?"

It took several years, but what Marty finally did about it was to hire Cyndy. Meanwhile Cyndy worked, unofficially, in her spare time, to design a plan for handling the kids whose lives had been saved, but who would return to a normal life only with long, careful restorative therapy.

There were similarities between the trauma kids and the congenitally disabled kids Cyndy had worked with; head-injured kids who regained consciousness often behaved strangely like retarded kids. They were loud, impulsive, hard to control. Some were echolalic: They would repeat words spoken to them but not originate any of their own. Others perseverated: They returned again and again to a single thought, a single idea, a single sentence. All of them showed deep emotional scars from their accidents.

But unlike retarded children, the head-injured children improved, slowly—agonizingly for their parents and nurses—but measurably. The return of consciousness did not mean the return of normalcy; the former often came quickly, the latter in slow, painful stages. Cyndy uses a measuring system called the Rancho los Amigos scale; it lists the types of behavior a child is likely to display as he regains his mental capacity. It is one of the first things she shows a child's parents, even before the child regains consciousness, to prepare them for what is to come. Only in the movies does the unconscious child open his eyes and immediately converse softly but intelligently with his parents. In the real world, the child is more likely to wake up screaming and cursing, as many a mortified parent has discovered. To Cyndy the curses are like music; they signal that the recovery process is working. From there, it is only a matter of time, and patience.

And with trauma kids, you never know where or when the healing will stop. That was the big difference with trauma kids, Cyndy discovered. They were unpredictable. Kids born with disabilities are fairly easy to evaluate, and it is possible to predict their lifelong limits with a fair amount of accuracy. With trauma kids you never know. They are so unpredictable that it is difficult to talk about norms and averages. In truth, there is no norm: If you set a mathematical norm, most kids will do better than the norm, while a few will do much worse. Even within wide limits of variability, it is nearly impossible to predict the long-range outcome of an individual trauma case. Some kids recover miraculously from horrible injuries; others lie comatose or heartbreakingly impaired. Often it is weeks after the accident before you know which is which.

It takes a special kind of temperament and a rigid and unswerving mental discipline to deal, day after day, with trauma kids and not go insane with grief. It is not possible to work with children and remain aloof from them; to work with them is to grow attached to them, to acquire an almost parental affection for them. This is particularly tough when you deal with trauma kids who, a few hours or days or weeks ago, were whole and full of promise. It is one thing to work with Down's syndrome kids, who were born that way; it is quite another to look at a child who, a short time ago, could reasonably have expected to become president, or to play in the World Series, or to find a cure for cancer, and realize that now the pinnacle of achievement for this child may be the ability to dress and feed himself. Parents at least can lie to themselves, refuse to accept a child's disability, fantasize that he will miraculously recover and still become president; rehab people have no such luxury. They must be realists, no matter how painful the reality.

Cyndy, like many of her colleagues in the rehab business, keeps her sanity by focusing on the small, positive issues instead of the greater, gloomy ones. She refuses to maunder over what the child might have been, preferring instead to be thrilled when the child begins to respond to voices, or to rejoice when he begins to speak.

The toughest part for Cyndy is that she is no longer a nurse. She is still an RN and has a master's degree to boot, but she no longer gives hands-on care; her job with the trauma service is purely administrative. She is in charge of rehabilitation planning and follow-up care for trauma service patients.

What that means in practice is that Cyndy spends a great deal of her time on the telephone, finding room in rehab centers for children who are no longer sick enough to stay at Children's Hospital but still too sick to go home. Likewise, she spends significant amounts of time badgering insurance companies, HMOs, and all levels of government to make sure that her trauma kids get every benefit to which they are legally entitled. Several federal laws protect the rights of handicapped persons; Cyndy knows them practically by heart and frequently flings them at foot-dragging bureaucrats.

On this particular Tuesday, she was especially furious with a particular health maintenance organization. HMOs are great cost-savers for people who have relatively minor injuries or illnesses; for major problems, they are usually inadequate. It is a problem inherent in the whole concept of HMOs; they were designed to provide health care at budget prices. Enough catastrophic cases will break the budget, and the HMO, so HMOs employ very strict gatekeepers, whose function, whether they admit it or not, is to deny care to people with serious long-term problems.

This places them squarely in conflict with people like Cyndy Wright. She has seen again and again the benefits of restorative therapy, and when the future of one of her kids is at stake, she will do instant battle. Her principal weapon is the telephone, with which she lobbies, harangues, blusters, fusses, nags, and shames reluctant providers into authorizing the rehab care her kids need. It is a constant problem; rehab is only beginning to be accepted as a worthwhile enterprise *within* the medical community; the insurance companies and HMOs that pay the bills will be even harder to convince.

In the long run, Cyndy will help make the case for all such kids; part of her job is to oversee a federally funded research project that will be gathering statistical evidence to show whether children with brain injuries benefit from intensive rehab therapy. On an intuitive level, on the level of individual case examples, the answer is that of course they do. But there are currently no statistical studies to prove it, and the lack of hard evidence has been used more than once as an excuse to write off a patient as being beyond all help. Ultimately, Cyndy's study will make it harder to deny rehab care to injured kids. For now, she still has to do battle.

Methodically, with the practiced patience of a rehab nurse, Cyndy made call after call. She called rehab centers, physicians, administrators at the HMO, the child's parents. After much wrangling back and forth, a compromise was reached: the HMO would pay for an initial round of rehab therapy, and if the child showed progress, then another round, and another, and so on. When she finally hung up the phone, Cyndy knew there would be a similar battle before each new round of therapy. That was fine; she'd fought that fight so often that she was getting very good at it.

She glanced at her watch, then quickly drained her coffee cup, gathered up a stack of file cards, and headed for Marty's office. On Tuesdays at 11:00 A.M. she, Heidi, and Marty conducted their own comprehensive bedside rounds. Marty is downright fanatical about making sure his trauma kids get complete medical care; Heidi and Cyndy share that fanaticism. Ordinarily, the code room and the intensive care unit are exclusively Heidi's dominion, while the general care floors and the outpatient follow-up clinic are Cyndy's. Once a week,

115

though, Heidi, Cyndy, and Marty take a tour of all the patient care areas, providing each other with instant second opinions to make sure nothing has fallen through the cracks.

Cyndy noticed the orthopedic gear over bed number three as soon as she walked through the doorway into the ICU; double ninety-degree traction is unique to broken femurs. Kids with broken femurs stay in the hospital a long time; Cyndy usually gets very well acquainted with them. There are also a lot of them; Kids who are old enough to run in front of cars are just the right height for the bumper to make contact with their upper legs. That is the easy part; all too often, the hood, and then the pavement, make violent contact with the child's head, and Cyndy finds herself with another long-term case.

Cyndy, Heidi and Marty stopped briefly at bed number one, where little Michael Jackson, his chest tube recently removed, complained bitterly about all facets of his hospital stay while a nurse and an orderly prepared him for transfer to 4-Blue. His punctured lung had, according to that morning's X-ray, healed completely. The plan was to keep him on 4-Blue for a day, just to be sure, and then send him home. The trio chatted and kidded with Michael long enough to turn his pouting into giggling, then moved on to bed number three.

David Myers Senior sat at the bedside, holding his son's left hand, staring absently into space. He looked up as the trio approached, nodded greetings to Marty and Heidi, whom he had already met, and shook hands with Cyndy as Marty introduced them.

"How's he doing,?" Marty asked Mr. Myers, nodding his head toward the boy but keeping his eyes on the father.

"There's not much change," Mr. Myers said slowly. "He had some rough times yesterday, but today everybody says he's stable." He picked up the boy's hand again, stroked it with a finger. "David," he said softly, bending over the bed. "David, can you say hello to these folks? Hey, picklehead! Say hello!"

Cyndy watched the boy's face intently. Had the eyelids fluttered just a trace? It was hard to tell. She glanced through the chart at the foot of David's bed, assembling a mental list of all the medications that were being used to keep the boy stable. The drugs made it hard to tell what was happening behind the closed eyelids. The boy might be trying to wake up, but the drugs would keep him quiet. For the moment, that was what he needed, but there would come a time when the crisis of his injuries would be past, and it would be time to think about leading a normal life again.

"PT/OT and speech consults," Cyndy said to her companions as they left little David's bedside. Physical and occupational therapy for unconscious patients is not a new concept; bending the limbs and flexing the muscles keeps them from tightening, from wasting, from becoming useless. Early bedside work by physical therapists can save hundreds of painful hours of rehab work later on. Speech therapy for an unconscious and intubated patient is a newer and more controversial idea, but one that Cyndy defends with equal fervor. Not all speech takes place with the mouth, she insists. Speech happens in the brain, and it uses the eyes and ears more than the mouth. Sometimes, to emphasize her point, she repeats the statement in sign language. Right now, the job of the speech therapist will be to watch David closely to see if he responds to sound at all, then to see if he responds differently to spoken words, and after that whether he responds differently to words spoken by his parents than to words spoken by strangers.

Inside little David's head, a badly swollen and bruised brain was struggling to right itself. So profound was the shock to that delicate organ that nearly forty-eight hours after the accident, the brain was still not capable of sustaining the little body without the help of a respirator and half a dozen powerful drugs. But with each hour that passed, dazed circuits would click back on, a few at a time, then a few hundred at a time, then a few thousand at a time, until finally the trillions of circuits that made up the brain of little David Myers had all either recovered or died.

Of all the specialized functions of the brain, hearing is one of the sturdiest. If David was going to recover at all, his hearing would be the first sense to return, and the speech therapists would be among the first to notice.

Fifteen _____

Public relations is not a particularly sentimental business, and Herta Feely would not describe herself as a particularly sentimental person. It came as something of a shock to her, then, the first time tears filled her eyes while she was trying to work.

It was supposed to be pragmatic work. The accident prevention campaign Herta was putting together had a number of highly pragmatic attractions. For one thing, it would draw national attention to Children's Hospital National Medical Center. For another, talking about children's injuries would lead naturally to the question of what happens when an accident is *not* prevented. Promoting the concept of children's trauma centers nationwide was, after all, one of the things Herta had originally been hired for.

As a means to an end, an injury prevention campaign had everything going for it. The statistics were very straightforward; Herta called up the National Safety Council and got a copy of *Accident Facts,* which is the definitive source of information when you want to talk about accidents. The statistics were sobering: Eight thousand children a year die in accidents.

Herta got out her calculator. Eight thousand a year was 666.66 a month. She punched in more numbers, then punched them in again. The numbers looked awfully high. Could 154 kids a week be dying from accidents? That was 22 a day, slightly less than one an hour.

Herta let out a long breath. She stared at the numbers she had written down. Every sixty-five minutes, somewhere in the country, someone's child died in an accident. She consulted *Accident Facts* again. Accidents were the leading cause of death among children; in fact, accidents killed more children than all other causes combined.

The shock grew even worse as she read on. In addition to the deaths, another fifty thousand children a year suffer some degree of permanent disability because of accidents. And even they are a tiny

118

minority of the *16 million* children who require medical attention because of injury each year.

From somewhere deep inside, a sense of outrage, a feeling of anger began to emerge. It was an anger she hadn't felt in a long while, not since her college days when she had marched against the Vietnam War. It was an anger that comes with the realization that lives are being wasted, thrown away, that the future is being squandered to no purpose.

She rechecked the numbers again. Could we be losing eight thousand kids a year, and crippling fifty thousand more, without so much as a whimper? My God, when we were losing that many soldiers a year in Vietnam, there were riots all across America. Could this be real?

Again, she turned to *Accident Facts.* The thousands and thousands of accidents were neatly broken down into categories. Automobile accidents, burns, falls, drowning, firearms, ingestion of poisons—preventable things. Easily preventable things. Eight thousand kids die each year due to carelessness? Fifty thousand kids are disabled by things we could have prevented? The numbers stared back at her, cold and unarguable.

What she needed was a campaign to wake people up, get them to think. Think safety belts. Think kiddie seats. Think about the cord dangling down from the ironing board. Think about barriers across pathways to danger. Lock up the drain cleaner. Lock up the firearms. Don't leave a kid unattended around water. Simple things, things everybody ought to know.

Marty had been right; most injuries were preventable. We use the word *accident* to deny responsibility. The first step had to be to educate grown-ups on child safety, make them aware of the problem. Probably half the fatal accidents in the country could be prevented. Imagine if you could save the lives of four thousand kids a year.

She toyed with the thought. Four thousand lives saved every year. Or, to be pessimistic, prevent 10 or 12 percent, and save a thousand lives a year. That would be a thousand kids a year who would grow up to lead healthy, productive lives because they didn't have a fatal accident. Nobody would ever know who they were, but the cold black numbers of the National Safety Council would show it, if she could reduce the accident rate.

A thousand lives a year. There was no doubt in her mind; with a proper budget and a free hand, she could mount a campaign that would save a thousand lives a year. A thousand kids, cute little kids like the ones crawling on the floor around the 4-Blue nursing station. The thought grew in her mind until she felt her eyes brim with tears. Something she'd known in the abstract for a long time was no longer abstract. This was what drove Marty Eichelberger; it was what drove all the members of the Children's trauma team.

To save even a single child was a great deed; to save hundreds, or thousands, was the stuff of dreams.

It would be the stuff of reality.

◆ ◆ ◆

Having picked a course to pursue, Herta found it almost absurdly easy to convince people of the worthwhileness of an accident prevention campaign. What proved difficult was convincing them to help pay for it.

Granted, much of the publicity would be free, in the form of public service announcements (PSAs) on radio and television. But someone had to produce the public service spots, send out the press releases, monitor the results. None of that was free. When Herta figured up her budget for a national injury prevention campaign, it came to several hundred thousand dollars.

She went back to the National Safety Council to ask their advice about where to look for funds. So persuasive was her pitch that the safety council chipped in a hundred and sixty thousand dollars, and not long after that, made an institutional decision to shift the safety council's own efforts toward accident prevention for children.

But except for that promised boost, the financial cupboard was dismayingly bare. Philanthropic institutions praised the idea and offered to contribute five thousand, or even ten thousand dollars. At that rate, Herta would spend all her time doing fund-raising instead of working on a campaign to prevent accidents. She brought in an enormous reference book that analyzed, among other things, the charitable donations of corporations and institutions and began laboriously paging through it, looking for a financial angel.

In the end it was the angel who found her, albeit indirectly. Herta was approached by a woman who wanted to produce a child safety videotape. The woman mentioned that the videotape would be used in a promotion by the Johnson & Johnson Health Care Company, the maker of Band-Aids.

Now that was a natural, Herta thought. What better tie-in to accident prevention than the people who made Band-Aids? The woman introduced Herta to her contacts inside Johnson & Johnson. At the same time, Herta's new friends at the National Safety Council passed the word along to their own connections inside J & J. Soon, Herta and Marty met with the top brass at J & J, making a pitch to Frank Ziegler, the president of the giant company's health-care products division.

Ziegler was astounded by the numbers, and shocked to learn that accidents killed more children than all other causes combined. More than anything else, he was shocked that he hadn't known about it before. If a top executive in a health-care-related business doesn't know, how in the world could you expect the general public to know? Ziegler promised he would pursue the matter.

Within two weeks, Johnson & Johnson decided to donate 4 million dollars—eight hundred thousand a year for five years—to the Children's Hospital accident prevention campaign. Herta had her angel. Together, they would save lives.

♦ ♦ ♦

No one, Herta included, anticipated the kind of response that the campaign kickoff generated. She had indeed pulled out all the stops; Surgeon General Koop, who by then had already become a legendary figure in the field of public health, agreed to be the spokesman for the National Coalition to Prevent Childhood Injury. President Reagan proclaimed Safe Kids Week at a ceremony in the Rose Garden at the White House. The story appeared in local newspapers, moved on wire services, and ran on national television. And the TV networks began broadcasting a pair of public service announcements on injury prevention.

The PSAs were carefully crafted to attract maximum attention in minimum time. The kids in the spots were cute, the message simple: Accidental injury is the leading killer of children. Call this toll-free number for a booklet that can help you prevent accidents.

When she began to plan the campaign, Herta had optimistically assumed that, over the course of the three-month push, they might get as many as twenty or thirty thousand calls requesting the booklet.

After ten weeks, when the phone calls topped seventy thousand, Herta phoned the networks and begged them to stop running the announcements. The campaign had been so wildly successful that it was in danger of going bankrupt. The networks complied, and the flood of calls tapered off, leaving Herta stunned, thrilled, and pushing the limits of her budget. Instead of a dozen local child-safety coalitions nationwide, there were fifty. Instead of a few thousand names, the mailing list was closing fast on a hundred thousand. She and Marty conferred with the executives at Johnson & Johnson; they agreed to increase next year's budget.

The injury prevention campaign had touched a nerve somewhere —it had illuminated, seemingly for the first time, a problem of such magnitude that everyone who heard of it was shocked, and moved to act.

In one of his many interviews on the subject, Surgeon General Koop observed that "if a disease were killing our children in the proportions that accidents are, people would be outraged and demand that this killer be stopped."

He was right, of course. When polio was killing children, mothers across America marched door-to-door and collected billions of dimes, and polio was cured. When boys scarcely past childhood were being wasted in Vietnam, people rioted in the streets until the killing was stopped.

How ironic, then, that without even a whimper we had allowed eight thousand children to die each year, and another fifty thousand children to be disabled, in accidents that should never have happened.

No, the amazing thing was not that Herta Feely had stumbled onto something bigger than the March of Dimes and the Vietnam War protests combined; the amazing thing was that no one had thought of it sooner.

Sixteen _____

Richard became almost like a mascot to the nurses on 4-Blue. He had nothing clinically wrong with him by the time he got there; his burns, which the burn unit nurses had kept swabbed with oils and ointments, had healed without the skin even peeling. When another burn case came in and they needed the bed, Richard got moved to 4-Blue. But Richard stayed in the hospital, tended by the 4-Blue nurses, for several more days.

Richard's only ailment at this point was social, not medical, and as a result, Children's Hospital was being forced to absorb all the costs of keeping him there. Insurance, including Medicaid, pays only for "medically necessary" hospitalization. Richard's tenure on 4-Blue could not in any way be justified as "medically" necessary.

Still, no one suggested that he should be released to his family. Indeed, within hours after Richard's admission to the burn unit, a judge had signed an order prohibiting the mother or her boyfriend from even visiting Richard without supervision, much less trying to take him home. Two days later, the police had arrested the boyfriend and charged him with criminal child abuse. There was talk on 4-Blue that the mother had agreed to cooperate with police and prosecutors, and might someday be able to reclaim her son, but it was more speculation than fact; the idea was to place distance between Richard and the troubles of his family, and the court injunction had done just that.

Richard, indeed, was blissfully oblivious to it all. He strolled the 4-Blue hallways, ranging sometimes as far as the 4-Green nursing station, demanding hugs of all his newfound nurse friends. Nurses at Children's Hospital like to hug kids in any circumstances, and Richard, now freshly barbered by a nurse who used to be a hairdresser, was almost unbearably huggable. Add to that the universal knowledge that Richard had been an abused child, and it was no surprise that

Richard got all the hugs he asked for and a few extra for good measure. Plus other goodies: The dieticians had threatened to start making nurses sign for every container of ice cream; Richard had gained weight during his hospital stay, presumably because of all the ice cream he had been able to wheedle.

The last couple of days, a gray-haired couple had come to visit Richard twice each day. They had brought him Christmas toys, children's books, and above all, by arrangement with the nurses, they had been the ones who brought Richard his daily ration of ice cream. They sat with him, hugged him, played games and sang with him, read aloud to him. After only a few sessions, Richard began to cry and pout whenever they had to leave.

The court-appointed foster parents duly reported all this to the 4-Blue nurses, who in turn notified the Social Work and Child Protection divisions, and the following day, Richard was discharged from 4-Blue and went home with his new family.

Seventeen

Three days before Christmas, after Mary Fallat and the residents had had their usual early-morning discussion at David's bedside, they removed David's endotracheal tube for what they hoped would be the last time.

David began to breathe, jerkily at first, but then more slowly, calmly, rhythmically. "That's very good, David," Karmy-Jones said, reaching out a hand to stroke David's shoulder. At K-J's touch, the boy's eyelids fluttered, and his breathing grew more labored, less rhythmic. As David tried to take deeper breaths, a harsh, rasping sound came from his throat. Karmy-Jones moved his hand away, and as David calmed down, the breathing became quieter.

Karmy-Jones hung around until Mr. and Mrs. Myers came back in. "He's breathing fine when he's calm," he told them, "but when he gets excited he starts gasping. This is a result of his having had a tube in his throat for three weeks. It should improve rapidly; if it doesn't, we'll have to consider doing a tracheostomy to give him a clear airway and give the upper part of his windpipe a chance to heal. Meanwhile, though, try not to do anything to excite him."

Mr. Myers nodded, walked to the bedside, and stroked the boy's upper arm. "David," he said gently, "everything's fine, David. Mommy and Daddy are here."

David immediately began a spasm of long, shuddering, gasping breaths, punctuated by attempts to cough. Mr. Myers stepped back from the bed, a look of anguish on his face. The harsh breathing continued, then slowly subsided.

"You see what I mean," Karmy-Jones said. His voice sounded tired. "He can breathe on his own, but when he gets excited he's not doing himself any good. We may very well have to do the tracheostomy, but for right now he's not in any danger. Let's give him a chance to improve on his own."

After Karmy-Jones left, Mr. and Mrs. Myers stood at the foot of David's bed, talking quietly to each other. David remained calm. Experimentally, Mrs. Myers walked up to near David's head and spoke quietly to him; his breathing became agitated. She backed away and he grew calm again. They tried playing a tape recording of music; he grew agitated at first, then calmed down. The nurse came to take his temperature; he grew agitated when the nurse put in the thermometer, and again when she removed it.

Mr. and Mrs. Myers held a bedside conference with the nurses and one of the ICU physicians. Each new stimulus excited David to the point that his breathing became labored, so the idea was to limit the stimuli. The nurses dimmed the lighting around his bed, drew the curtains partway. Mrs. Myers drew up a stool and sat near the bed, but not directly at the bedside. Another long vigil had begun.

◆ ◆ ◆

On the morning of Christmas Eve, Marty Eichelberger scheduled David for a tracheostomy. There was no particular urgency about it, only resignation. After three weeks of being stretched around the hard plastic tube, David's throat was so inflamed and swollen that his vocal cords had become paralyzed, and for all anyone knew, they were permanently damaged. His bruised lungs had healed, but in doing so they had secreted a great deal of thick liquid that congealed inside them. If David had a normal airway, he'd be able to cough up the phlegm, but since he couldn't cough, he had to be suctioned out periodically. Suctioning had to be done with a flexible plastic tube, which of course irritated the windpipe even more. It was an impossible situation; David could get enough air to lie quietly, but any time he grew excited, the damaged windpipe could not accommodate the increased demand, and David's breathing would become harsh and labored. It had not improved in the two days since the breathing tube had come out.

The trauma team's only choices were to put the tube back down David's throat for another few weeks, which would guarantee that his vocal cords would be destroyed, or to cut a hole in his throat and install a bypass route to his lungs, a tracheostomy. They chose the latter.

Before anesthesiology became sophisticated enough to use safely the endotracheal tube, which follows the natural airway to the lungs, tracheostomies were much more commonplace, and that simple hole in the throat, just below the Adam's apple, has saved many a life. Today, the objective is to avoid all those things by rapidly teaching the patient to breathe again on his own. Usually it works. This time it hadn't.

Patricia and David Myers stood quietly at little David's bedside. They couldn't talk to him, or play tape recordings for him, or hug him as they wanted to; all those things caused him to gasp for breath. So as they stood at the bedside, they simply held hands and said a brief prayer that the surgery would go well and that it would help little David. When the orderlies arrived to take David to surgery, they went back to the ICU waiting room and prayed again.

The orderlies made no attempt to unhook David from his orthopedic gear; they simply disconnected the electronic monitor leads, hung the IV bags from a pole attached to the bed, and wheeled the entire bed out of the ICU and down to surgery. In the operating room they were met by an anesthesiologist who injected a cocktail of drugs into David's IV line and, when he went limp, put an endotracheal tube back down his throat. She did not attach him to a respirator; instead she used a black bag rhythmically to force oxygen-rich air into the boy's lungs.

With David anesthetized, the nurses and orderlies went to work on the orthopedic gear. After three weeks, David's broken legs had healed to the point that the traction could be discontinued in favor of casts, but manipulating the legs would still have been painful had David not been anesthetized. With the ropes and pulleys disconnected, David looked even smaller, more fragile and vulnerable. At the foot of the bed were David's three toys, including the stuffed bear Nancy Reagan had given him. "Isn't that cute?" the circulating nurse said, picking up the bear. As soon as she moved the bear, it responded with an electronic voice. "Oooh, hug me, hug me!" the bear said in baby talk so realistic that the anesthesiologist gave a little shriek and looked sharply at her patient before she realized the words hadn't come from him.

Drs. Eichelberger and Karmy-Jones arrived wearing OR gear but still not scrubbed. They surveyed the scene, moving close to the bed as the orderlies pulled it alongside the OR table. Six sets of hands lifted the small body onto the operating table; an orderly held his legs, keeping them bent at the correct angle, while Marty and one of the nurses stuffed rolled blankets under his knees to keep the legs bent.

Even that gentle manipulation worked loose the fragile clots around the steel pins in his legs, and tiny drops of blood seeped out around them. The OR team didn't notice, though; they were already busy arranging little David's head. Another blanket roll went under his neck, so that his head was bent back, neck fully extended. Before doing the tracheostomy, Marty planned to explore the boy's lungs.

A bronchoscope is simply a long, polished stainless steel tube with lenses at both ends. That tube fits inside a slightly larger tube, which can be connected to a respirator. By maneuvering the tubes, Marty could visually explore David's lungs. From listening to David's lungs with their stethoscopes, the doctors knew that David's lower lungs, as they had healed, had become clogged with mucus. The ICU nurses had been able to suction most of the secretions out of his upper lungs, and that was plenty for David to breathe with, but now Marty intended to clean out the lower lobes too. With a tracheostomy, David would find it much easier to cough, but this would give the boy a head start.

Marty fiddled with the eyepiece at his end of the bronchoscope, checking adjustments and alignments. "Is he paralyzed yet?" he asked the anesthesiologist without looking at her.

"Yep," the anesthesiologist replied. "Ready for you. You ready?"

Marty didn't reply. Instead, he drew up a stool directly at the head of the bed, so that little David's face, tilted far back, pointed directly at his chest. Karmy-Jones, standing directly beside him, used a flat metal instrument to hold David's mouth open while Marty, in a single deft move, took out the plastic ventilator tube in David's throat and replaced it with the bronchoscope tube. Immediately the anesthesiologist connected her black bag to the new tube.

"Is he ventilating?" Marty asked.

"Not yet," the anesthesiologist replied.

Marty pushed the tube farther in. "Now?"

"Not yet."

Farther. "Now?"

"That's good. Perfect."

"Okay. Gimme a wet sponge," Marty said to a nurse. The nurse handed him a wad of dripping gauze. Marty carefully lifted the tube, which rested on David's teeth, and put the gauze sponge under the tube. No sense chipping a tooth; the boy had enough things to worry about already.

On the inside, David's windpipe was a zebra pattern of bright red and bright white stripes, extending far down toward the lungs. Inflammation, severe inflammation, covered in places by white secretions. The breathing tube had kept David alive for three weeks, but at a cost.

A branch appeared in the path; Marty jinked the tube to the left and proceeded down the left bronchus and into the upper lobe of David's left lung. "Upper lobe looks pretty good," he commented. "Looks like they got most of it upstairs." Marty continued squinting into the eyepiece, his head moving forward as he maneuvered the tube through passageway after passageway, navigating his way to the lower lobe. "Now. There. C'mere and look at all this junk," he said to Karmy-Jones. K-J bent over and squinted through the eyepiece, then another resident did the same. The surface of the lung was covered with lumps of yellowish-white.

"That's what gives you the pneumonia," Marty said. "That's what gives you the collapsed lungs." As he spoke, he withdrew the inner tube of the scope and, working blind, threaded a flexible plastic suction tube back in its place. When the suction tube reached its destination, the clear plastic filled with globs of the mucus. Marty twirled the plastic tube to reach as much of the stuff as possible. Still not satisfied, he removed the suction tube. "Let me have some saline," he said to the nurse. Holding the syringe at the top of the hollow tube, Marty squeezed out two cc of clear liquid, let it run down the long tube into the lung. Then he slid the suction tube back down again, and again the tube turned gray as more goop came bubbling out.

"Looks pretty grungy, doesn't it?" Marty commented to Karmy-Jones. "This is what he gets from lying on his back for three weeks."

The process took nearly an hour. With infinite patience, Marty explored each segment of the lower left lung, cleaning as he went. When he finally was satisfied with the left, he withdrew the tube nearly a foot, maneuvered into the right bronchus, and repeated the same painstaking process for the entire lower right lung. It was slow going; there was so much gunk in some places that it obscured the view, and Marty would have to stop, clean off the viewing tube, clean the area around the tip of the outer tube, and then continue his journey.

"Okay, that's it," he announced finally, adding, to the anesthesiologist, "ready?"

"Yes," she said.

"Okay, here goes." With one long smooth motion, Marty slid the entire bronchoscope assembly out of David's throat. A muscle twitched on the side of the throat, but David, paralyzed by the anesthetic, did not breathe. The anesthesiologist held David's mouth open while Karmy-Jones used the suction tube to remove the small amount of gunk that had come out with the tube, then reinserted an endotracheal tube into David's windpipe. Each new intubation worsened the inflammation in David's throat and vocal cords, but like everything else in medicine, it was a trade-off. With the tracheostomy in place, David's throat could heal at its own pace.

Marty and Karmy-Jones retreated to the scrub sinks outside the operating room while the scrub technician, the circulating nurse, and the anesthesiologist got David ready for the surgery. The nurse scrubbed his throat several times with brown antiseptic liquid; Marty and K-J returned, dripping hands held high, and quickly donned their scrub gear and sterile gloves. Then they did another series of antiseptic scrubs along the full length of David's neck. They quickly applied a series of sterile drapes, and in moments, only a single patch of skin was visible in the harsh blue-white OR lights. The skin still glistened with brown antiseptic.

Marty and K-J took up positions on opposite sides of the table, Marty on the right, K-J on the left. With the blunt tip of a hemostat, Marty pointed to a spot on the exposed neck, then to a second spot. K-J drew a scalpel blade between the two points, and a layer of bright white fat appeared, then began to turn red. The operation had begun.

"A little deeper," Marty said. K-J drew the scalpel down the incision a second time. Drops of blood began to appear on the exposed flesh, and Marty clamped hemostats over the larger ones. "Coagulation," he said quietly, and K-J applied an electric cautery to the smaller bleeders. Blue sparks crackled from the coagulator blade, burning shut the small blood vessels. A faint smell of smoke permeated the operating room.

Layer by delicate layer, K-J worked his way deeper into David's neck, tunneling toward the windpipe. Marty spoke quietly, sometimes almost inaudibly, naming each new layer as K-J exposed it, caught it with tweezers, and divided it with scalpel or scissors.

"Watch out for the blue there, watch out for the blue there," Marty repeated again and again to K-J. A large vein, dark blue in color, was clearly visible on one side of the incision. "You hit that, we'll have a mess on our hands. Watch out for the blue there."

Finally, a pale bluish white surface appeared: the trachea. "Stop right there," Marty said. "Let's back out and look for bleeders." The two surgeons stopped, reconnoitered, and coagulated two tiny spots where blood still oozed into the wound. Meanwhile, the scrub tech opened a sterile package and dumped a white plastic tracheostomy assembly into a stainless steel bowl. The trach tube was bent so that the airway part could extend an inch or so down the lower part of David's windpipe, then terminate in a round plug the size of a quarter that would protrude out the front of David's throat.

"We'll want three-oh silk," Marty said to the scrub tech. The tech tore open two sterile envelopes, snapped suture clamps over the two curved needles, and handed one to Marty, one to Karmy-Jones. The trachea was tough and rubbery; both surgeons had to push to get the needle through and plant the sutures, one on either side of where the incision would be made. With the black thread dangling from either side, the trachea was ready.

Holding the scalpel just between his fingertips, K-J made a quick vertical slice along the surface of the trachea. Frothy blood immediately foamed out of the incision. "Suction, please," Marty said. "Make it a little longer," he added to Karmy-Jones. K-J flicked the scalpel, and the incision grew. More blood foamed out.

"Ready?" Marty said to the anesthesiologist.

"Ready."

"Okay, go," Marty said. Grasping the two sutures, he held the incision in the trachea wide open. The endotracheal tube was clearly visible through the blood that continued to froth out. Karmy-Jones, holding the trach assembly in his right hand, began pushing the curved end of the tube into the incision.

"Pull," Marty said to the anesthesiologist. Reaching underneath the surgical drape, the anesthesiologist began to slide the tube out of David's throat. "Good, good, good," Marty encouraged. "She's pulling good."

Inside the respirator a pressure sensor noticed the sudden drop, and an alarm began to sound. The surgical team ignored it. "Okay," Marty said to Karmy-Jones, "slide forward now, slide forward, forward—we're in."

The respirator alarm continued to beep. "Let me get in there for a second," Marty said, reaching under the sterile drape to grasp the respirator hose that the anesthesiologist was pushing toward him. He grabbed it, connected it to the newly installed tracheostomy tube. "I'm connected," he reported to the anesthesiologist. "Is he ventilating? Can you ventilate him?"

"Sounds good," the anesthesiologist replied.

"We got a good seal," Marty said. "He's ventilating."

Marty and K-J removed the sterile drapes, wiped the area clean with gauze pads. The incision in David's throat had already closed tightly around the plastic trach tube; there was no bleeding. David's chest heaved rhythmically. When the anesthesia wore off, David would be breathing through a new and improved airway, and his tortured throat would finally be left alone to heal. Marty stripped off his gloves and sterile gown, tossed them in a nearby hamper. "I'll go talk to his mom and dad," he announced as he strode out the door.

Eighteen _____

Nightmare Monday began as a gorgeous spring day, the kind of warm, sunny day that kids dream about when they grow tired of snow and ice. It was a school holiday, which made the playing that much more fun. Even though it was too early in the year for swimming, Anna Foster put on her favorite pink bathing suit to remember the feel of it. A trace of chill lingered in the air, so she pulled on a yellow T-shirt over the suit. Later, when she went outside to play with Susan, another ten-year-old who lived nearby, she added a pair of high heels to her costume. Larry, her eight-year-old brother, tagged along.

The day grew prettier by the hour, as only a Virginia spring day can do. The Fosters were newly arrived Texans, and since they had moved into the house in February, they had seen nothing but snow and ice followed by slush and mud. Now the ground was nearly dry, the grass had begun to turn green, the dogwood trees were sporting delicate white blossoms, and over the long weekend the Fosters had decided that perhaps the East Coast was not such a bad place to live after all. This day bolstered their opinion; it was an incomparably lovely day.

As the children ran outside, their mother, Joan Foster, warned them to stay in the yard and thought no more about it. The Foster home was perched on a hillside, separated from the main road by a quarter mile of sloping gravel driveway. The children had plenty of room to play in without ever coming near the highway. Mrs. Foster stayed indoors to do laundry. Tom, at sixteen the oldest child, stayed indoors, too, for the more serious business of playing electronic games on the family's Apple computer. It was a slow, leisurely day—a perfect holiday.

Outside, Anna and Susan, with Larry in tow, paraded around the yard playing fantasy games. Presently they climbed into the back of the family pickup truck, which was parked near the top of the long

133

driveway. The pickup had a wooden bed that had worn smooth with years of use, and was an ideal place to conduct a make-believe tea party or to take a make-believe train ride. The children jumped up and down in the truck bed, shrieking and giggling.

When the truck abruptly began to roll backward down the drive-way, it took only a brief, breathless moment for all three children to realize that something was terribly wrong. Anna screamed "Jump!" but waited until Larry had bailed out over the left side and Susan over the right before she herself jumped off the back. The truck, still gathering speed, knocked Anna down and rolled over her, then clat-tered and bounced down the slope, swerved off the driveway, and plunged tailfirst into a brushy ravine where it finally stopped. There was a sudden silence.

Larry stumbled when he landed but immediately scrambled to his feet and turned just in time to see the truck run over his sister. Her body twisted as the wheels passed across it, but then she lay still, facedown at the edge of the driveway. There was a growing spot of red on her forehead. Susan and Larry both stared openmouthed for several seconds; then Larry began to scream and raced for the house.

Inside, Mrs. Foster and Tom were still in the basement of the house, but they heard the door slam, and then suddenly Larry was at the top of the stairs, gasping and sobbing, begging them to come quickly—the truck had rolled down the driveway and was in the ditch. Mrs. Foster and Tom stood up and walked toward the stairs. Then Larry added that the truck had run over Anna.

Mrs. Foster was nearest the stairway, but Tom was faster, and by the time she was halfway to the first floor he came bounding past her, taking two steps at each stride, and raced out the front door. Tom reached Anna first and knelt beside her briefly. Then, as Mrs. Foster arrived, Tom stood up and sprinted back to the house, shouting that he was going to call an ambulance.

Anna was still facedown on the gravel. Blood covered her left eye and streamed across her face. There were tread marks across her bare legs. Mrs. Foster knelt for a moment, then simply sat down in the driveway next to her daughter. She had no idea what she should do next. She had never taken so much as a first aid course; none of the children had ever even been near a hospital before. But when Anna roused and began trying to move, some instinct stirred in Mrs. Foster, and she put a gentle hand on Anna's shoulder. "Don't try to move, honey," she said. "You stay right where you are until the ambulance can get here."

Inside the house, Tom dialed 911 and, with scarcely controlled impatience, gave the ambulance dispatcher directions for how to get to the Foster house. "Hurry," he added. "She's not moving. She's hurt bad."

Tom raced back outside. "Stay with her a minute," Mrs. Foster told him. "Don't let her move around." Then she got up and ran for the house.

Mark Foster worked for a home builder, and he spent so much time driving from job site to job site that the company had installed a mobile phone in his car. Now his wife punched out the numbers, hoping to catch him between projects. She did. "Where are you?" she asked.

"Out on Route Fifty," he said. "What's wrong?"

His wife explained briefly. "The ambulance isn't here yet. I guess they'll take her to Chesapeake. Why don't you go straight there?"

She hung up the telephone, looked out the window, and saw that the ambulance had not arrived. Patience, she told herself. We live a good distance from town. I'm sure they're hurrying. But it was hard not to panic. She felt bewildered, helpless. If only she knew a little first aid. . . .

Blankets. They always covered accident victims with blankets. She'd seen it on television, and a few times in person. She went to a closet, found a woolen blanket, and headed outside.

Anna hadn't moved. Tom was sitting on the ground beside her, talking to her. "Here, honey, this will keep you from getting too cold," she announced as she spread the blanket over Anna. She hoped it was the right thing; even though it was not a hot day, she could see that Anna was sweating a little.

"How do you feel, honey?" she asked.

The reply was soft, muffled. "It hurts to breathe," Anna said. "I feel like I can't get my breath."

Mrs. Foster turned to Tom. "Go call the ambulance back. Tell them she's having trouble breathing. Ask them please to hurry."

◆ ◆ ◆

The ambulance came slowly down the winding highway, the driver obviously looking at street numbers on the mailboxes. Tom and his mother stood and waved their arms, and the ambulance driver accelerated up the gravel driveway, stopping a few feet away from the spot where Anna lay.

"She's having a hard time breathing," Mrs. Foster said. "Please hurry." The medic stepped out of the ambulance carrying a backboard, a neck collar, and a stethoscope. The driver and medic crouched beside Anna. One held her head while the other grasped her hips, and together they gently rolled her over and onto the backboard. Seconds later the neck collar was in place. While the driver ran back to the ambulance, the medic began listening to her chest with his stethoscope.

The driver returned carrying a green oxygen tank and a box of supplies. The medic dug into the tool kit, brought out a green plastic face mask, and attached it to the oxygen cylinder. He slid an elastic band around Anna's head to hold the mask in place, then opened the valve. The escaping oxygen made a hissing sound, and the clear plastic turned foggy. The medic turned to Mrs. Foster. "What's her name?" he asked.

"Anna."

The medic bent close to the girl's ear. "Anna, can you breathe any easier now?" he asked.

Anna tried to nod, but the neck collar held her head still. "Yes," she whispered.

"That's good. We'll get you to the hospital in just a minute. First, I'm sorry, but we've got to cut that pretty bathing suit off so we can see if you're hurt anywhere."

Anna tried to nod again, then whispered, "Okay."

With a few strokes of the scissors the pink bathing suit and yellow T-shirt were in shreds. The medic pulled the clothing away, replaced it with a white bed linen as he scanned the tiny body for obvious wounds. He found none. He listened again with the stethoscope, frowning. Breath sounds on the left side were definitely fainter. He put down the stethoscope. "Anna, I want to count your ribs. You tell me if anything hurts. One . . . two . . . three . . . four . . ."

"Owww!" Anna winced as he reached rib number five. That settled it, the medic thought. Broken rib, punctured lung. Maybe more.

"Let's go," the medic said to his partner. While the second man ran to the back of the ambulance and unlatched the rolling gurney, the medic made a quick inspection of the cut over Anna's left eye, satisfied himself that it didn't include the eye itself, and taped an antiseptic-smeared gauze pad over it. By that time the driver had arrived with the gurney, and the two men lifted the backboard onto it. They buckled Anna into place with seat-belt-like straps and whisked the gurney into the back of the ambulance.

"What hospital are you going to?" Mrs. Foster asked.

"Chesapeake, right now, because it's close," the medic answered. "If they find anything serious, they may want to fly her up to Children's Hospital in Washington."

"How do I get there?" she asked.

Tom interrupted the conversation. "You ride to the hospital with Anna," he suggested. "Larry and I will follow you in the car." He pointed to the brown Volkswagen Rabbit still parked in the driveway. Tom had turned sixteen only a few months before and was proud of his new driver's license.

Mrs. Foster turned to the ambulance medic. "Is that okay?" she asked.

"Fine," the medic answered, but then added to Tom, "Don't try to follow right behind us," he said. "That's dangerous. Just drive normally, take your time, and you'll get there quick enough. Okay?"

"Okay," Tom said over his shoulder, heading for the house.

The medic and Mrs. Foster climbed into the back of the ambulance with Anna, and the driver maneuvered the vehicle back down the sloping driveway, red-and-white lights flashing. When he reached the street, he turned on the siren and sped away.

Tom and Larry ran through the house quickly, checking to be sure all the doors were fastened, then jumped into the Rabbit. The Rabbit was the family's car, but it was the one Mr. and Mrs. Foster particularly liked Tom to drive, because it has unusual seat belts. They are anchored just behind the gearshift, but the other end is fastened to the door, so that when a passenger gets into either front seat and closes the door, he is automatically belted in. It was a handy system; it made it impossible to forget to wear a seat belt.

The quickest way to get to Chesapeake Hospital from the Foster house is straight up U.S. Route 1, a wide four-lane road that, in the days before interstates, was the principal north-south highway on the East Coast. Now it is a wide, highwaylike road that looks dangerously like a highway but is crisscrossed by intersections, some with traffic lights, some without. The ambulance driver kept his vehicle near the center of the road and kept his siren wailing. Even so, he slowed down as he neared each intersection; he'd had too many near misses at Route 1 traffic lights.

In the back of the ambulance, Mrs. Foster watched as the medic expertly started an IV line in Anna's right forearm. "Just in case she's bleeding inside," he explained. "That'll help us keep her stable."

Despite the traffic hazards, the ambulance covered the seven-mile distance in little more than seven minutes. A nurse and a doctor greeted them outside the emergency entrance, then helped unload the gurney and wheel it inside into an examining room.

The physician spoke heavily accented English and often had to repeat his questions, but he quickly established that Anna's left side hurt, and he noticed that she was pale and having trouble breathing. During a brief examination, the doctor also noticed that Anna tended to flinch when he pressed on her abdomen. That, too, was a bad sign. People with internal injuries behave that way. The physician was beginning to suspect that this was a case he should consider transferring to Children's Hospital.

Before he phoned Children's, though, he wanted a little more information. There was a portable X-ray machine nearby, so he ordered films of Anna's neck and chest. While the X-ray technician was getting set up, he quickly drew a blood sample, instructed the nurse to install a Foley catheter, then started a second IV line in Anna's left forearm. Two IVs were better than one, if Anna proved to have internal bleeding.

The Foley was also a quick way to diagnose serious internal injury, and the doctor was relieved when it produced clear urine with no visible sign of blood. While he waited for the lab and X-ray results, he busied himself by unbandaging, cleaning, and rebandaging the cut over Anna's eye.

When the X-rays arrived, the doctor took one look at the chest film and reached for the telephone. The girl clearly had partial collapse of the left lung; this was a case for Children's.

"How bad is the pneumothorax?" the physician at Children's asked. The doctor described what he saw on the X-ray and read the results of the lab studies. "I think it would be wise to go ahead and put in a chest tube before you transport her," the Children's physician said.

The doctor protested. He said he would prefer that the procedure be done at Children's, but the physician on the other end of the line was firm. It needed to be done now. The physician described the procedure in detail, noting the anatomic landmarks, the things to watch out for. The doctor at Chesapeake hung up the phone and stalked off in search of instruments.

While the Park Police helicopter was on its way to Chesapeake Hospital, the emergency room doctor assembled his instruments, drafted a nurse to help, and successfully installed a chest tube in Anna's left side. When it didn't seem to help as much as it should, the doctor ordered a second chest X-ray and discovered that the tube had gone past the main air pocket. He pulled the tube back a short distance, the tube filled with pink air bubbles, and Anna agreed that now it was easier to breathe. Anna seemed so calm and tolerated the procedures with so little complaining that the doctor secretly worried; hurt children are not supposed to be so grown-up about it.

Anna's father arrived with a police escort of sorts; when he got to the city limits, he had flagged a police cruiser and asked for directions to the hospital. "Follow me," the policeman said and sped off with Mr. Foster in pursuit. When he arrived, the emergency room doctor had already talked to Children's, had already put in the chest tube, and the Park Police helicopter was already on the way. Mr. Foster just had time to go see his daughter before she left for Children's Hospital in Washington.

◆ ◆ ◆

After they unloaded Anna, the ambulance crew waited around awhile, hoping to get their neck collar and backboard before they had to take another call. The medic wheeled a fresh IV set from the charge nurse to replace the one he had used for Anna, and while he was at it, picked up a few extra bandages as well. Ambulance companies are chronically short of funding; hospitals help subsidize them by replacing whatever supplies they use on an incoming patient.

Midafternoon is shift-change time around hospitals; the evening shift is from 3:00 to 11:00 P.M., and the ambulance medic was surprised to see one of the ER nurses come bustling in the door nearly fifteen minutes after her shift was scheduled to begin. As she took off her sweater and stowed her pocketbook, she apologized profusely to the nurse she was due to relieve. She had left her house on time, she said, but there was a bad accident down on Route 1, and traffic had just been totally snarled for the last half hour.

"Did you see what ambulance company was there?" the medic inquired from the other side of the nursing station.

"There wasn't an ambulance there," the nurse replied, "and I'm not sure why. One of the cars, a little brown Volkswagen Rabbit, was just smashed to pieces. I'd be amazed if someone wasn't hurt."

"Brown Volkswagen Rabbit?" The medic did a slow double take. He and his partner stared at each other. No. It couldn't be. Or could it? Where were those boys, anyway?

"We gotta go," the medic said. "We'll be back." The two men ran out the door, leaving their supplies behind.

◆ ◆ ◆

Mr. and Mrs. Foster waited tensely at Anna's bedside while the helicopter was summoned. There was not a lot to do; they tried to make small talk with Anna, but the oxygen mask she still wore made conversation difficult, and even though she remained alert, she seemed little inclined to chat. The nurse who had just come on duty introduced herself, and with a brief apology to Anna drew another blood sample. It was important, she explained, to have very fresh lab results to send with Anna on the helicopter flight.

While the nurse was with Anna, Mr. and Mrs. Foster slipped out into the hallway. How in the world were they going to find their way to Children's Hospital? They had just begun to learn their way around their own suburb; neither of them knew anything about driving in downtown Washington. Mark suggested calling a friend who worked at the construction company, who was a native of the area and could drive Joan to the hospital. He would have to find his way with a map, Mark said; he explained that on his way there, he had phoned his mother in Dallas and she was already on her way to Washington. Her plane would land late that evening, and he would stay around to pick her up, then come to the hospital with her. Joan agreed that it had been a good idea to call her; for the next few days at least, they'd need an extra grown-up around to take care of the boys. Joan looked at her watch again; the boys were certainly taking their time. Maybe they were stuck in the traffic jam she'd heard the nurses talking about.

The doctor approached Mr. and Mrs. Foster with consent forms. One was for the chest tube procedure that he had already done; the other was a consent to transport Anna to Children's Hospital. The doctor explained that Children's was a much larger facility, with pediatricians on duty around the clock and all the resources to give

Anna the best possible care. The nurse, who had finished reexamining Anna, stopped and joined the conversation. "Don't worry about a thing," she told Mrs. Foster, putting a hand on her arm. "Children's is a very good hospital." The doctor nodded assent.

There was a commotion behind them, and the emergency room doors swung open as a gurney rolled through. Mrs. Foster turned, saw the face of the medic who'd taken care of Anna, and smiled a greeting at him. The man didn't smile back; the look on his face was strange, grim. He stared at Mrs. Foster for a long instant, then dropped his eyes. Joan Foster followed his gaze down to the gurney. Her son Larry lay strapped to it, his eyes wide with fright. Mrs. Foster put a hand to her mouth, felt her knees weaken. One nightmare had become two.

Nineteen _____

Before Gerry Pratch came on the scene, Tom McGinley had given lots of talks, lectures, and slide shows about how to take care of an injured child, but there had been no formal curriculum, no course outline, no real way to measure how well the students were learning the system.

Gerry, fresh from graduate school, took on all those jobs simultaneously. First, she had to learn the Eichelberger method of taking care of injured kids. That part was easy; Gerry knew pediatric nursing from her previous five-year hitch at Children's; the trauma protocols were logical and straightforward, and they were already in writing. Gerry's first job was to take the "field provider" information and put it into writing. The result was a slim paperbound volume, coauthored by Gerry and Marty, setting down the procedures that ambulance crews should follow in dealing with an injured child. Today the book is distributed nationally.

As she developed the text, she also taught it to ambulance medics from all around Washington and its suburbs. The medics were a bright bunch, full of questions and war stories; the curriculum grew with each new course Gerry taught. The DeVore Trust, impressed with the early results, extended the grant to give Gerry more time to train more medics.

The training program had, in a roundabout way, identified a significant blind spot in modern trauma care: The field medics, without exception, had not been properly trained in pediatric trauma. And if this was true in Maryland, the birthplace of modern emergency medicine, what must prehospital care be like in Missouri, North Dakota, or Oregon?

But a year after she came to Children's, and after dozens of training sessions with medics, Gerry concluded that she had taken on an impossible job. There was simply no way one person, or even one

team, could train every ambulance medic in the Washington Metropolitan Area alone, let alone anywhere else. There simply were too many of them. What she needed was a program to train teachers.

The U.S. Department of Health and Human Services and the Department of Transportation agreed, to the tune of several hundred thousand dollars. The training program established Children's as the nationwide pediatric training center for paramedic instructors. Under the terms of the grant, Children's was to recruit and train at least two instructors for each of the fifty states. The instructors got all-expense-paid trips to Washington, and an intensive week-long course covering every facet of pediatric trauma care. In between lectures the medics would spend time in the emergency room, the ICU, and the burn unit. After five short days, they would return to their home states loaded with information, ready to begin training local paramedics in how to deal with pediatric emergencies.

In the beginning, Gerry's classes had spread the word to perhaps a dozen field medics at a time. Now, each class would, in the end, reach hundreds.

And Gerry no longer taught the classes. After the birth of her first child, she cut back her schedule to half-time, and now she spends her workdays preparing new grant proposals, and articles for publication in professional journals. The HHS/DOT grant provided salary money for two full-time people to run the training program.

◆ ◆ ◆

For Jane Ball and Eliane Runion, the pediatric EMS course is a grueling time, a week of fourteen-hour workdays sandwiched between two travel-agent weekends, as they shepherd a dozen paramedic instructors into town, oversee their week-long training regimen, and bid them bon voyage the following weekend.

By all accounts, the training program has been a winner. The large map of the United States in the instructors' office has sprouted a proud crop of colored pins—two at least, and sometimes more, in every state. The instructors have gone back full of facts and enthusiasm, and the files that Jane and Ellie keep on each state's progress are filled with letters describing successful local courses taught by the newly trained instructors and attended by dozens of local paramedics.

The course has filled in a valuable chink in the educational armor of most paramedics. Virtually all field-care training in emergency

medicine concerns how to treat an injured adult. Out of a hundred or more hours of training, pediatric trauma care gets perhaps an hour or two.

It is a serious gap. Children are different, very different. First and most obviously, they are smaller. A blood-pressure cuff designed to work on an adult is far too large to take an infant's blood pressure. Yet for the medic in the field, blood pressure is one of the most important pieces of data when trying to decide how badly a patient is hurt.

Children are not just small; they come in all different sizes. A four-year-old is too big for an infant blood-pressure cuff but not big enough for an adult one. Likewise, children of different ages will have different-size blood vessels, an important consideration if a child is bleeding severely and needs intravenous fluids. So in addition to a range of blood-pressure cuffs, the field medics need an array of different-size needles and tubes.

And what about drugs, medications? Obviously you don't give an infant an adult's dose of painkiller, but how much do you give? If you give intravenous fluids to combat blood loss, how much do you give? An adult quantity would drown a child. If the child isn't breathing and you have to breathe for him or her, how much pressure should you use? The pressure you would use for an adult could burst an infant's lungs.

And those are just the highlights. There are hundreds more differences, large and small, between an injured adult and an injured child. On the first day of the course, the dozen paramedic instructors receive an enormous blue three-ring binder. Among its voluminous contents are charts, descriptions, and rules of thumb for determining size-appropriate therapies for injured children.

The binders will largely remain closed during the week-long course; printed information can be reviewed back home. The trip to Washington, D.C., is not for reading; it is for a total-immersion introduction to injured kids—which is, ultimately, an introduction to kids in general.

"Look at it through the child's eyes," Cyndy Wright tells the class early on the first morning of the course. "Everything is different. First of all, everything is up. You have to look up to see everything. You're little; everything around you is big. Then you ride your tricycle out into the street where you're not supposed to be, and you get hit by

a car. The car is huge, the people who stand around you are huge. Then an ambulance comes, and maybe a police car and a fire engine, and they're even bigger.

"Then out of the back of this very large ambulance comes a stretcher, and big orange boxes, and all sorts of strange-looking stuff, and more big people. They hold you down, put a hard collar around your neck so you can't move your head, strap you onto a backboard so you can't move anything else—you're three and a half years old. Would you be terrified by now?"

Heads nod around the room.

"Now you can't *not* do all those things just because they may frighten the child," Cyndy goes on. "Obviously, you have a procedure to follow to minimize a child's injury. But you can try to minimize the terror at the same time.

"Talk to the child. Here at Children's Hospital we have one nurse in the code room whose job is to talk to the child, keep them calm, keep them oriented. Do that in the ambulance, too, if you can. Explain things to them; talk to them on their level, but talk to them the whole time."

"That's if you can stop them from crying," observes one of the medics.

"Why do you want to stop them from crying?" Cyndy asks. "If you're three and a half years old and you get hit by a car, you're *supposed* to cry. That's the appropriate response. What you ought to worry about more are the ones who don't cry.

"When I walk through the emergency room and hear kids screaming, that's—well, it's not okay, but I know that it's an appropriate response. The ones I worry about are the chronic asthma kids, for example, who have learned that it doesn't do any good to fight because they're going to get that IV anyway. Kids cry by instinct; they have to *learn* not to cry, and a child who learns that at too early an age is someone to worry about."

The talk lasts an hour. Cyndy shows slides, tells war stories, hands out photocopies of favorite cartoons to illustrate her points about kids. Kids are not miniature adults but little people in their own right, Cyndy says, and if you remember that and deal with them on their own level, you can make an awful experience a little less awful. It is an easy, friendly lecture, a good show opener.

After Cyndy comes Hal Lipton. Cyndy spoke of dealing with the

145

child; Hal's topic is dealing with the family. Hal is the head of the Social Work Department at Children's Hospital; as Marty Eichelberger oversees the care of the injured child, Hal Lipton oversees the care of that child's injured family.

"What do you say to the parent or parents at the scene? There are no 'right words,' " Hal tells the group. "I don't have any lists of 'right things to say.'

"I can tell you one thing *not* to say; don't ever tell a parent you know what they're going through unless you've been through it. In fact, don't ever tell them anything that's not completely true, even if you're only trying to comfort them. So there's *one* 'right thing to say' —the truth is the right thing to say."

Hal pauses, surveying the group. "Then there are times when you have to know what not to say. Imagine you arrive at an apartment to find a two-month-old infant with a broken leg. The mother tells you the child crawled out an open window and landed on the leg."

"Two months?" asks one of the female instructors, incredulously. Hal nods, smiling.

"Two months. And you know full well that a two-month-old child can't crawl out a window. Now, what do you say to that parent?"

"I don't think you should make any accusations right there," says one. "Ask as many questions as you can, try to remember as many facts as you can, and when you get the child to the hospital you can let the authorities know what you found."

"That is precisely right," Hal says. "You don't want to be judgmental. You don't want to let your own feelings, no matter how strong, interfere with the job you're there to do. The best thing you can do for any parent in any circumstance is to treat their child efficiently, professionally, rapidly, compassionately. They may not show it at the time, but they will appreciate that more than anything else."

Hal's talk lasts an hour, with Hal throwing out increasingly complicated scenarios, all of which have actually happened, some once or twice, some more often. Soon the medics are adding their own war stories, and the roundtable runs well over into the coffee break.

Already the medics are hooked. This is the real stuff; these are scenes they've all confronted themselves, in the field back home. The polite expressions they arrived with have been transformed into eager, sharp-eyed interest. This is good, practical, nuts-and-bolts stuff they are getting, and they are ready for more. For the next four-and-three-quarters days they will be soaking it up as rapidly as the Children's Hospital staff can dish it out. By the time they board their flights home, they will be full of missionary zeal, ready to spread the word in their home states.

Which is exactly what Marty Eichelberger, and the DeVore Trust, and later the Departments of Transportation and Health and Human Services had in mind.

Twenty

Things were very confused for several minutes after Larry Foster came in the emergency room door at Chesapeake Hospital. As they pushed the gurney into the examining room the ambulance medics assured Mr. and Mrs. Foster that their oldest son, Tom, was okay. He had bit his lip in the accident, they said, but they had examined him at the scene, and he appeared to be fine. Larry had been walking around when they got there, too, but had complained of chest and abdominal pain. They had brought him in as a precaution.

"But what happened to them?" Mrs. Foster demanded.

"Somebody ran a light right in front of them," the medic replied. "It wasn't their fault; they had the green light. They're both very lucky they were wearing their seat belts; the Rabbit's a real mess."

"How will Tom—"

"The police said they'd drive him home," the medic said, anticipating the question. "He's fine, really."

While they spoke, the ambulance medic, the driver, and Mr. and Mrs. Foster all followed the stretcher into an examining cubicle. The same doctor who, an hour before, had been examining Anna now pulled back the sheet and began examining Larry. When he pressed on Larry's abdomen, the boy grimaced and drew back. "Guarding," the movement is called in medical jargon. A bad sign; when a patient is guarding his abdomen, it means something hurts inside. The specter of internal bleeding haunts every accident room. The physician moved to a telephone, called the X-ray department.

Mr. Foster stood at Larry's side, squeezing one of his hands, murmuring encouragement to him. He left only when the portable X-ray machine was wheeled alongside Larry's bed. Then Mrs. and Mrs. Foster mustered in the hallway for a quick conference. The family friend had arrived, and they quickly agreed that she and Mrs. Foster should head for Children's Hospital. "You go stay with Anna," he said, "and I'll stay here and look after Larry." The two women left, and Mr. Foster headed back to Larry's bedside. The emergency room doctor was standing there, examining the X-rays.

"I'm worried that he has some internal bleeding," the doctor said. "I want to do some additional X-rays using a special dye that will show us if he's bleeding anywhere inside." The doctor offered Mr. Foster a consent form; he signed it, handed it back. The doctor nodded to a pair of orderlies, and they began wheeling Larry's bed out of the emergency room, toward the X-ray department.

◆ ◆ ◆

When Mrs. Foster arrived at the Children's Hospital emergency room, the place was a madhouse. There were people everywhere, crowded into the bus-station-style waiting room, sitting in the hallways, milling around. They all had children with them, and most of the children were crying. Shrieks of hysteria emanated from the double row of examining rooms as doctors and nurses cleaned wounds, drew blood samples, gave shots, or simply tried to examine frightened children. It was a mob scene.

Hesitantly, Mrs. Foster approached the central nursing desk, caught the eye of one of the nurses. "I'm Anna Foster's mother," she said. She started to explain that Anna had been brought in by helicopter, but the nurse stopped her.

"She's here," the nurse said. "They just took her up to X-ray. She's awake and talking to us. She's a real sweetheart." The nurse pointed to a pair of elevators. "Take one of those elevators to the second floor. X-ray is right in front of the elevator doors."

Mrs. Foster remembers being impressed that, in all the bedlam, the nurse knew immediately who Anna was and, more important, where she was. In fact, the nurse she spoke to had, minutes before, been in the code room with Anna. But any other nurse at the desk would have known about her as well: Cases that come in by helicopter are high-priority cases, and so are their families.

The elevator doors opened at the second floor, and Mrs. Foster stepped out cautiously. To her left, a small clump of people in white lab coats stood just outside a doorway. They noticed her immediately. "Are you Anna's mother?" a woman asked, walking toward her. Mrs. Foster nodded. The woman held out her hand. "I'm Heidi. I'm the trauma coordinator. Anna's in there," she said, nodding her head toward the doorway. "We're getting ready to do CAT scans." As

149

Heidi talked, she guided Mrs. Foster toward the doorway. "We can squeeze in here for just a minute before they start. Anna!" she called out as they entered the room. "Look who's here!"

Anna lay on a table-height platform in front of a huge metal donut. The size of the machine made Anna appear especially tiny and frail. The nurse had put web straps across her hips and shoulders to keep her from accidentally moving during the scans, but her hands were free. She squeezed her mother's hand with a firm grip and smiled at her.

"How are you doing, honey?" Mrs. Foster asked.

"Okay," Anna said softly. "Everybody's been real nice. Where's Daddy?"

"Grandma's flying up from Dallas to visit you," Mrs. Foster answered. "He's got to pick her up at the airport." She hesitated, wondering whether now was the time to tell Anna what had happened to Tom and Larry. Heidi solved the dilemma for her.

"Anna," Heidi said, "we have to wait out in the hall now, while they do the X-rays. We'll be right outside, and as soon as they're done we'll be back. Remember to lie real still, okay?"

"Okay," Anna said. Heidi guided Mrs. Foster outside. Just beyond the doorway, a man in an immaculate white lab coat approached them.

"This is Dr. Eichelberger, the director," Heidi said as the man held out his hand. "Marty, this is Anna's mother."

"Hi, nice to meet you," Marty said casually. Then, looking her directly in the eye, he added, "How're you doing?"

"Well, it's been quite a day," Mrs. Foster answered with an audible sigh. "My youngest son was hurt in a car wreck on the way to the hospital to see Anna. He's at Chesapeake, and my husband's with him. Anna doesn't know about that yet." She shook her head. "I guess I'm okay, but I sure wouldn't want too many more days like this one."

Dr. Eichelberger whistled softly. "I guess not," he said. "We'll find you a phone so you can check on your son in a minute," he continued, "but first let me bring you up to date on Anna.

"Right now the worst problem seems to have been the broken rib, which caused one lung to collapse part of the way. The way you manage that is to put in a chest tube and remove the air that's outside the lung; that lets the lung fully inflate. The lung usually heals itself within a day or two, and then we can take out the chest tube. They put the chest tube in back at Chesapeake Hospital, and when she got here we double-checked it. It's working fine; we think we have that under control.

"The reason we're doing a CAT scan is because she has some tenderness in her abdomen." Marty pointed to his own left side. "Right about here, where the spleen is located. Plus, we did find evidence of blood in her urine, and because of those two things we're a little concerned that she might have an injured spleen. The CAT scans will tell us that.

"If she does have a splenic injury, there is a remote possibility we'd have to do surgery, but the chances are we wouldn't. Kids are wonderful; most times, if you just leave 'em alone they'll heal. What we would do is watch her very closely for a couple of days to give the spleen a chance to heal itself. We don't want to do surgery unless we absolutely have to.

"The cut over her eye is superficial. It bled a lot, so it must have looked real bad, but there's no danger at all from the cut. As soon as we rule out all the more serious stuff, we'll get a plastic surgeon in to close that wound. I can't say whether there'll be a scar, but I would wager there won't be. Our plastics guys are good.

"As soon as we finish doing the CAT scans, we'll move Anna to our intensive care unit so we can keep a close watch on her. You'll be able to stay with her in ICU; in fact, we encourage parents to spend a lot of time with their kids. We think it's good for 'em."

Marty shifted, looked around. The briefing was clearly finished. "We need to find you a telephone," he said, half to himself, half to Heidi. "Where's a telephone around here?"

"The cafeteria?" Heidi prompted.

"Yeah, the cafeteria," Marty agreed. He looked at Mrs. Foster. "There are phones all over the cafeteria. Dial nine. You've got some time before they finish here. Oh, and the coffee's good, too."

♦ ♦ ♦

At Chesapeake Hospital, little Larry Foster grew bored with all the waiting. He fidgeted on the gurney, he hummed and sang a little, he talked to his father about cherished television programs and even dozed occasionally. The nurse, a sharp-featured woman with dark hair, came around every few minutes to check his heart rate and blood pressure; she bantered with Larry in a motherly way and quickly made friends with him.

151

Getting acquainted with an insider seemed to diminish Larry's fright; when they moved him into the X-ray room his eyes got very wide, but the nurse stayed at his side and held his hand, and he grimaced but did not cry out when they used a huge syringe to inject X-ray dye into his arm.

While the films were being developed, the two attendants pushed the gurney back down the hallway to the emergency room. Shortly after that, the doctor approached Mr. Foster.

"We see on the films evidence that your son has an injured spleen," the doctor said. "This is potentially a very serious problem. If the bleeding were to continue or get worse, he could go into shock. We think it will probably be necessary to take him to surgery to repair the spleen. But first we want to do a diagnostic procedure here to see if we can determine how bad the bleeding is."

The only infallible test for internal bleeding is peritoneal lavage, better known as the belly tap. Sterile liquid is flushed into the abdominal cavity, then drained out. If it comes out pink, there is internal bleeding. The only hitch is that gaining access to the abdominal cavity requires minor surgery. The doctor told Mr. Foster he'd need to sign a consent form.

Mr. Foster wavered. "I need to think about this for a minute," he said, looking first at Larry, then at the doctor.

"I understand," the doctor said. "I'll be out at the main desk."

Mr. Foster stood at the foot of Larry's bed. His mind raced. Larry lay on the bed, humming quietly to himself, looking contented and healthy. According to the doctor, there was a time bomb inside the boy's belly that could go off at any instant. Mr. Foster's mind rebelled at the thought of sending Larry into surgery, but on the other hand . . .

The nurse appeared at Larry's bedside, blood-pressure cuff and stethoscope in hand. "Hi, Larry," she said cheerfully. "Time to squeeze your arm again." Larry dutifully held out his arm. As she applied the cuff, she looked at Mr. Foster. "I just phoned Children's," she announced. "They said your daughter's doing fine."

"That was real nice of you to do that. I appreciate it," Mr. Foster said. "I just wish I knew what to do now. You know what they found here?"

The nurse nodded, the disk of her stethoscope pressed into the crook of Larry's arm while she squeezed the bulb of the blood-pressure device.

"I don't know what to do," Mr. Foster said. "I don't know what to do. I can't even talk to my wife; she's forty miles away in another hospital."

"Children's is a very good hospital," the nurse said thoughtfully. "A very good hospital."

"I hate to send Larry into surgery without being sure about it. But if I wait for a second opinion, and something happens—" He stopped. The nurse looked at him. "What should I do?"

The nurse looked away. "I can't make recommendations to you. I'm not a doctor. But you know, Children's is a very good hospital."

"If his spleen really is injured, and anything happens to him, I'd—"

"Children's," the nurse said, looking Mr. Foster straight in the eye, "is a very good hospital."

Mr. Foster's look of puzzlement vanished as it dawned on him what the nurse was saying. "I see," he said. "Yes, I see. You know, you're absolutely right. Thank you. Thank you more than I can possibly tell you."

Mr. Foster walked out of the room, and up to the emergency room desk. The doctor was there, writing in a chart. After a moment he looked up.

"I want Larry moved to Children's Hospital," Mr. Foster said.

Twenty-one _____

The day after Christmas, they moved little David Myers out of the intensive care unit. With the tracheostomy in place, there was no longer any reason to keep him in a high-tech environment; what medical care he would need now was routine. What he needed more was good nursing care and rehabilitation.

The general surgical wing of Children's Hospital is on the fourth floor. The floor is divided into zones, each identified by a color: green, blue, orange, or yellow. The surgical rooms are on 4-Blue. One of the nurses took David's parents on a brief tour just before the transfer.

Mr. and Mrs. Myers were especially grateful for the change; at Children's Hospital, general care rooms are private rooms, and each room, in addition to the hospital bed, has a sofa bed where a parent can sleep. Parents are not simply allowed to stay overnight, they are encouraged to do so.

The drain on Patricia and David Myers had been astronomical. Both had missed enormous amounts of work; all their vacation time was gone, and while both their bosses had been sympathetic and supportive, there were rules to be followed, and the time they took now was put down as leave without pay. The handsome savings account, the money they had worked so hard to put aside, was vanishing at a distressing pace; there was plenty of insurance to pay for David's hospital care, but after that, what?

Even in the chaos, a sort of routine had emerged. Mr. Myers had arranged to work evenings, Mrs. Myers mornings, so that one of them could always be at David's bedside. Mrs. Myers's mother had flown up from Georgia, and she kept the household from disintegrating; she cooked, tidied the apartment, spent time at the hospital. Soon the three of them began to rotate overnight duty at the hospital. For the first time in a month, Mr. and Mrs. Myers were able to spend time together, away from the hospital.

154

They spent a great deal of time worrying about what would become of their son. He had not progressed according to expectations, and as a result the doctors had again and again scaled back their expectations. In the face of ever-more-gloomy prognoses, though, Mr. and Mrs. Myers tried hard to remain optimistic.

After all, they reminded each other, just when the doctors had been predicting that he would never wake up, he had begun to respond to their voices. That had been a wonderful moment; both of them often talked to David as they sat at the bedside, but for interminable days, David showed no sign that he heard them. Then, one afternoon, Mr. Myers leaned over and whispered a word that, before the accident, had always been guaranteed to make little David giggle. "Hey, pickle-head," Mr. Myers said.

Little David grinned.

Mr. Myers jumped as though a jolt of electricity had stung him. He looked around for the nurse, caught her eye, motioned to her. She bustled back to the bedside. David lay still, looking asleep. "Pickle-head," Mr. Myers called to him.

David grinned.

"David, that's wonderful," the nurse cooed, stroking his head. "You're getting better, aren't you?" Again, the grin, but Mr. Myers didn't see it; he was wiping tears from his eyes.

After that, there had begun to be tiny signs of improvement, just enough to keep Mr. and Mrs. Myers from losing hope. At the same time he began to smile, he also began to frown, even to cry. His broken legs still swung in traction then, and though the bones had begun to knit, moving the legs was still painful. David's face would cloud up, his mouth contorted as though he were trying to say "Owww," and sometimes tears would leak from his closed eyes.

It wasn't constant; David faded in and out. Sometimes he seemed only a hairsbreadth away from waking up; other times, nothing could rouse him.

And that was the status of the patient that Eve Zimmerman received, the day after Christmas, on 4-Blue.

Children's Hospital, like many other hospitals, assigns a "primary nurse" to patients who are likely to be in the hospital for more than a day or two. The primary nurse becomes that patient's personal in-house advocate; the primary nurse, for example, is responsible for designing an individual nursing care plan for her patient, and enforc-

155

ing it. The primary nurse is the family's main contact, and the main conduit between the family and the rest of the hospital staff. Often, the nurse's relationship with the family grows into an almost familial bond; nurses at Children's Hospital get lots of Christmas cards.

Most of all, the primary nurse is the patient's primary bedside care provider. Other nurses will come and go from shift to shift; a primary nurse may have other duties as well, but when she is on duty, the patient is hers, and she must look after all his routine and nonroutine needs.

For David Myers, the list of needs was a long one. He had a fresh tracheostomy, which was, after all, a sort of wound—a hole in his throat. The wound could become infected; Eve would have to watch for the telltale inflammation and apply antiseptic creams as a preventive.

David's legs no longer swung in traction; the orthopedics people had replaced the weights and trapezes with a plaster cast that extended from David's hips to his feet and kept his legs bent at precisely calculated angles, so his broken femurs could continue to heal. The cast roughly doubled David's body weight, which made turning him a great deal of work. The cast also kept his lower body immobile, which meant he had to be turned more often so that he wouldn't develop bed sores.

The tracheostomy in David's windpipe was connected to a canister arrangement on the wall that bubbled oxygen-rich air through plain water to humidify it so it wouldn't cause the trachea to dry out and become inflamed. The canister had to be refilled with water every few hours; if it ran dry, David could develop a raging sore throat.

Then there were the routine needs of an unconscious patient. David wore diapers, and they had to be changed periodically. He was being fed high-calorie nutrients that dripped from bags that had to be changed, through a nasogastric tube that had to be checked. There were orders to take his vital signs—temperature, pulse, blood pressure, respiration rate—every four hours. The patient had to be bathed, his bed linens changed, his teeth brushed, a thousand little details. Eve worked constantly, steadily, from the start of her shift to the finish, and often well beyond. She went home bone-tired every day.

Most important of all, she talked to David, cooed at him, stroked his head, wiggled his toes, patted his shoulder. Unconscious patients who are left in quiet isolation tend to remain unconscious; Eve's friendly voice and gentle touch were probably the most valuable parts of David's medical care.

David was not strictly unconscious; he smiled and frowned in response to voices. He made faces and cried noiselessly when he felt pain. Sometimes he even opened his eyes, but the eyes didn't track. They were the eyes of a blind person.

The physical and occupational therapy specialists came in and out and seemed satisfied that David's overall muscle tone had stood up well despite a month in bed. The dieticians stopped in from time to time, saw a well-nourished and healthy boy, and from time to time made minor adjustments in the high-calorie liquid diet that continued to drip directly into David's stomach through the tube in his nose. The speech-hearing specialists watched him closely and were cautiously encouraged by his progress, though they pronounced it unusually slow. At the therapists' recommendation, Mr. and Mrs Myers bought several cassette tapes of children's stories and bought extra batteries for the cassette player. When nobody felt like talking, they would play a story tape.

There were days, now, when Mr. and Mrs. Myers were absent from the room for several hours at a time. Eve had encouraged them to go back to work. Eventually, she told them, David would need a place to come home to; they would be doing him no favors if they neglected everything simply to be at his bedside. Besides, David needed to learn to do without one or the other of them in constant attendance; sooner or later, he'd be going to a rehab center, and there'd be hours, perhaps even days, between visits.

But while his parents began to spend slightly less time at the hospital, David never wanted for company. Besides Eve, he had another new companion, Jim Riddell, child-life specialist.

Child life is one of those marvelously attractive concepts that, unfortunately, is confined mostly to dedicated children's hospitals. Many hospitals have pediatric sections, but few of them have an entire department whose sole mission is to make life more pleasant and more nearly normal for the hospitalized child.

Jim Riddell is a sort of year-round Santa Claus. To the outsider his job appears to consist almost entirely of bringing toys into children's hospital rooms and helping them play with the toys.

What shows only if you read the child's medical record is that Jim is actually a trained observer, and that the toys are carefully calibrated for age-appropriateness. Children with severe, debilitating injuries tend to regress intellectually and developmentally while they are recovering; the invisible part of Jim's job is to provide yet another stimulus to the child's developmental recovery, and yet another assessment and opinion of just how well that development is progressing.

The first time Jim visited little David Myers, he brought a small hand bell, a miniature version of an old-fashioned school bell. He pressed David's fingers around the handle, then waved David's hand around to make the bell ring. David grinned.

"That's good, David," Jim said. "Now ring the bell again." Nothing.

"C'mon, David, ring the bell." Nothing.

"Hey. Boo-boo. You. David. Make noise. Ring the bell." Slowly David rocked his hand from side to side. The bell clanked dully. A grin spread across David's face, and he raised the bell in the air and shook it, slowly, awkwardly, but with a clear ringing sound. The grin grew to a wide-open-mouthed expression of joy.

"Attaboy, David. You show 'em." Jim's grin matched David's. He had read all the gloomy predictions in David's medical record. According to the specialists, David would be blind, mute, crippled, and severely brain-damaged. Watching the boy joyously ring the hand bell, Jim wasn't so sure. Don't write this child off yet, he thought to himself.

As the days stretched into weeks, Eve repeatedly brought up the question of where Mr. and Mrs. Myers wanted to send little David for rehab therapy. The choices were fairly limited; there was one center in Virginia, one in Delaware, and one in Baltimore—the John F. Kennedy Institute at Johns Hopkins. Eve discussed the relative merits of the different centers with Mr. and Mrs. Myers, and they dutifully toured the Virginia and Baltimore centers.

But they seemed oddly reluctant to make up their minds. It was as though, after all this time, the hospital routine had become such a part of their lives that now it was normal, and to change it would be to upset things.

Eve talked to Leslie Strauss, the social worker whose territory included the ICU, and who had become friendly with Mr. and Mrs. Myers during David's long stay there. The two of them then called Cyndy Wright into the discussion.

Their consensus was clear: David's parents, without realizing or understanding it, had become psychologically dependent on the hospital and its staff. It made a certain amount of sense; after all, the hospital had saved their son's life and had taken charge of his life for all these many weeks; it was only natural that a sort of bonding process had begun to take place.

There was a danger in that process, too: Terminate the bond too abruptly and you create hurt, then anger and frustration. Neither Mr. and Mrs. Myers, nor indeed their son, needed any additional stress right now. Even this long after the accident, they were still treating not just an injured child but an injured family.

The best way to defuse things was to let the decision be made in a large, neutral forum, a patient care conference. Cyndy got on the phone, and midway into January, Eve, Cyndy, Leslie Strauss, and several of David's attending physicians sat down at a conference table with David's voluminous medical record—and David's parents.

"We've done as much as we can do for him here," Cyndy explained to them. "His major injuries are all healed; he's not in any medical danger any longer. What he needs now is constant intensive therapy, and we're not equipped to give him that here. We were very good at fixing his immediate injuries; that's what we do best here. Now he needs to be in a place that specializes in restorative therapy, to give him the best possible opportunity to get better."

Mr. and Mrs. Myers nodded. One by one, the doctors and nurses added their own recommendations for rehab therapy. Marty Eichelberger wasn't there, but the argument presented to the parents was the same argument Marty had used again and again, the one that had never failed: *It's for the kid; this is what the kid needs.* In the end, the parents had no choice but to pick a rehab center. They picked the Kennedy Institute. The doctors and nurses agreed on a date for moving David to the institute, and that was that. Mr. and Mrs. Myers went back to their son's room, vaguely unhappy yet somehow satisfied that this was the right thing to do.

Twenty-two _____

Medic One bucked and wailed through the streets of Washington, D.C., as Van Coppedge, the driver, frantically tried to shave extra seconds off the ride to Children's. In the back, paramedic John Proper struggled to keep his balance, bracing himself against one side of the ambulance as he bent over the patient, pushing rhythmically against her chest.

His patient was a fourteen-year-old girl; she had been standing in a schoolyard with several friends when a gang of youths rode by on motorcycles. For reasons nobody quite understood, one of the motorcyclists pulled out a pistol, and as they passed, he fired into the group of children. The girl, Tanessa Starnes, collapsed on the sidewalk.

By the time Medic One arrived on the scene, Tanessa had no pulse. She was unconscious, breathing only in brief agonized gasps. The medics tore open her blouse, saw the tiny entrance wound on the left side of her chest, and began to move very rapidly. One started an intravenous line while the other quickly zipped Tanessa into MAST trousers. They hoisted her onto their gurney, raced back to the ambulance, and—less than five minutes after they had arrived—were speeding toward Children's.

Coppedge grabbed the microphone of his two-way radio. "Medic One, Children's" he said.

"This is Children's. Go ahead, Medic One."

Coppedge took a deep breath. "Medic One is en route, teenaged girl, gunshot wound left chest, no pulse, CPR in progress, ETA four minutes."

There was a brief silence. "Okay, Medic One, four minutes. We'll be ready."

The radio operator at Children's Hospital was grabbing for the phone with his left hand even before he released the radio microphone button with his right. "Trauma stat, ER, CPR, now." The communications operators know when to fudge on the ETA. This was not a case where anyone could afford to dawdle.

The trauma service office is only a short walk from the radio room, so Heidi was one of the first to arrive. "Gunshot wound to the chest," the operator told her. "Full CPR. No pulse. Bad one. ETA about two minutes."

Heidi's mind raced. For a pulse to disappear so fast could only mean one thing: that the bullet had penetrated the heart. When that happens, the tough membrane around the heart rapidly fills with blood, and the pressure of all that blood prevents the heart from beating. The condition is called cardiac tamponade, and there is only one way to treat it: heart surgery, right in the code room.

This might have been one of those rare cases when Marty Eichelberger himself would have crossed the threshold of the code room, except that Marty was out of the building. Heidi grabbed a phone, dialed the surgery offices. "Where's Kurt?" she demanded. Kurt Newman, the newest member of the permanent surgical staff, had completed his chief residency the previous year; for two years before that, he had been a trauma team coordinator.

The secretary explained that Dr. Newman was in the neonatal intensive care unit, performing minor surgery on a baby. Heidi cut her off, dialed the NICU.

"Dr. Newman," one of the nurses called out, "It's Heidi. She says it's very important."

Newman, in full scrub gear, glared over the magnifying loupe spectacles he had to use to find a preemie's tiny blood vessels. "Does she know I'm scrubbed?" he said.

"I told her. She says it's very important."

Newman handed scalpel and hemostat to the resident assisting him. "It's all yours," he said, stripping off his surgical gloves. Kurt had worked with Heidi both inside and outside the code room. When Heidi says it's important, it's damn well important. He put the phone to his ear, listened for a few seconds, then headed for the emergency room at a dead run.

The sixty or so seconds between the time Newman arrived in the code room and the time his patient arrived gave the surgeon scant time to organize his team. "Open the thoracic tray," he ordered the ICU nurse. "You," he said to the surgical resident, "start doing cutdowns. Don't diddle around putting in IVs; put in the biggest tubes you can find and start squeezing. Where's the blood?" he said looking around.

"Two here, more on the way," a nurse answered.

"Okay, you," he said, looking at the ICU resident, "give bicarb and epinephrine boluses right away; then we'll start a cutdown in the other arm, too." A cutdown is the fastest way to get blood into a patient. Slice through the flesh, expose the largest vein you can find, puncture it and slide a tube into it. Tie a suture around it, and you have a high-volume pathway into the circulatory system. With enough cutdowns, you can counteract even massive bleeding.

"Can we get another OR nurse down here?" Newman said. "I'm gonna need a scrub nurse, I'm almost sure." Outside the code room, the assistant director of nursing reached for the phone.

The double doors burst open and three medics clattered in, two dragging the gurney, one holding an IV bag. "We got a heartbeat back just now," one said breathlessly, "but it's real erratic." The gurney slid up beside the code room table. The girl was on a backboard; it bounced as eight people half slid, half tossed it onto the table.

The girl's chest heaved erratically, the breaths harsh in her throat. At the head of the table, the anesthesiologist slapped two heart monitor disks onto the already-exposed chest. The bullet wound was a tiny, dark, puckered hole. There was deceptively little blood.

"I'm not getting a pulse," nurse-left called out, while resident-left speared a vein and injected heart drugs. "No pulse at all."

"You," Newman said, pointing at John Proper, the paramedic, "We need you to do CPR." He turned to the anesthesiologist. "Are you going to intubate her?"

"I think that would be a good idea," the anesthesiologist replied, reaching for a laryngoscope. The paramedic stepped up to the table, near the patient's right shoulder, leaned forward, and began pressing rhythmically on the center of her chest. Resident-right, meanwhile, had moved to the girl's groin and was probing with a scalpel for the large saphenous vein.

Newman, standing on the left side, watched the heart monitor. There was electrical activity, but no pulse, no regular heartbeat, no effort by the heart to pump blood. There was only one thing do to: cut.

Grabbing a bottle of dark brown antiseptic liquid, Newman sloshed a great deal of it onto the girl's chest and left side, swabbing it around with gauze pads. Then he turned to the scrub nurse, who had just arrived and was now standing beside the tray of chest instruments. She held out an opened package of sterile gloves, and Newman jammed his hands into them. There was no time to scrub, no time to drape the patient. He grabbed another antiseptic-soaked gauze pad, swabbed the left side again, then reached for the scalpel.

A thoracic scalpel is a large-bladed instrument, and Newman bore down hard as he cut through fat and gristle between the fifth and sixth ribs. There was no bleeding; the patient had no blood pressure. There had not even been time to administer an anesthetic, nor was there a need: The patient was already unconscious. Indeed, for all practical purposes the patient was already dead.

Resident-right finished installing a second cutdown in the girl's groin, attached a bag of whole blood to it, and handed it to a nurse. "Squeeze," he commanded. There were now two IV lines and two cutdowns in place; the girl had already received nearly an entire unit of whole, unmatched type O blood. A blood-bank technician rushed in with two more.

Newman continued to cut, widening the already-gaping wound between the girl's ribs. Down through layer after layer of muscle, each slice of the knife deepening the wound until finally he penetrated the chest cavity, where the heart and lungs are located. As soon as the knife broke through, blood began to pour out. As he widened the incision, the trickle turned to a flood and dark, partly clotted blood slopped out onto the floor, soaking his shoes and socks.

"Wow," said the nurse squeezing blood into the saphenous veins. There must have been tremendous pressure inside the chest cavity; at the moment Newman opened it, she felt the blood bags in her hands soften as the back-pressure fell. She squeezed harder. "Need another one," she said over her shoulder. One bag was already empty.

Newman probed the wound with a gloved finger. A retractor was spreading the incision wide, but it still was not big enough to get a hand in. "Scissors," he said, holding out a hand. The nurse handed him a pair of heavy-gauge shears. Reaching the scissors into the upper part of the incision, he began snipping the wound open. When he came to a rib, he grabbed the scissors with both hands, squeezed, and snipped right through. He tested the incision again. This time his hand fit inside.

"Okay, when I tell you," he said to the paramedic, "stop your CPR for just a second." He was squatting now, looking in through the wound, at the pericardium, the tough membrane that surrounds the heart. The pericardium was dark blue and swollen, filled with blood. He had to open it to let the blood out, but he had to be careful not to cut the heart muscle at the same time. "You got any good forceps, with teeth on them?" he asked the scrub nurse.

"Try this," she said, handing him a long hemostat.

Newman looked at it, frowned. "That the best you've got?" he said.

The scrub nurse rattled instruments in the tray. "Looks like it," she said.

"Okay," he said with a shrug. It took several frustrating tries to get a purchase on the pericardium with the hemostat, but finally the teeth grabbed and locked. He pulled back, creating a tiny tent of membrane. Then he reached in with scissors, sliced open the tent, and more blood gushed onto the floor. "Okay, stop CPR," he ordered. The medic backed away.

Working quickly now, he sliced open the rest of the pericardium, then reached inside. The fingers of his right hand curled around the soft, quivering heart muscle. Gently, cautiously, he squeezed, then relaxed, squeezed, then relaxed. The heart responded with a spontaneous contraction.

When the heart contracted, Newman felt a warm sensation against his palm. He moved his hand slightly, exploring the heart's surface until his fingertips located the hole, near the top of the heart. Sliding his thumb over that hole, he began feeling around toward the back of the heart, and quickly located the exit wound, covering that one with his middle finger. The heart muscle contracted again.

"I'm getting a pulse," nurse-left called out excitedly. "I'm getting a pulse!"

"We're not done yet," Newman said. "I've got my fingers over two holes in the heart."

◆ ◆ ◆

During the daytime Maggie Huey, the emergency room nursing supervisor, is the gatekeeper of the code room. She is the person who stands outside the door, next to a wall phone, controlling who goes in and out, and relaying information to and from the trauma team, over the phone. She also coordinates the activities of all the people outside the code room, the extra hands that make it possible for the inner core team to have whatever resource it needs.

164

This day, the frantic needs of the code room team had drained off all her people so that, when the surgical resident announced that they needed more blood, there was no one left to send for it. "Watch the phone," she called to Heidi, as she set off down the hallway in search of more help. Heidi, with the ease of many years' experience, moved into position beside the phone, which already was ringing again.

"Code room. Heidi," she said crisply into the receiver.

On the other end of the phone was a highly agitated chief technician from the blood bank. "You're using up all my unmatched O blood," the chief technician said frantically. "I've got to have a sample to type and cross-match, and I've got to have it *now*. If you wait until you've replaced her entire volume, I'll be testing my own blood. This is crazy."

Heidi looked through the doorway into the code room. You think it's crazy, you ought to be down here, she thought. As she watched, Dr. Newman dropped a bloody scalpel into the instrument tray, and began spreading open the girl's chest with his hands while a resident tried to work a retractor into place. Near the girl's right shoulder the ambulance medic, standing on a footstool, leaned heavily on the girl's chest as he continued to apply CPR. On the heart monitor behind the bed, fluorescent lines jumped crazily, but there was nothing that looked like a heartbeat.

"I see your point," Heidi said after a long pause, "but things are, uh, pretty busy right now." She thought a moment. "The real problem, though, is that she doesn't have any blood pressure. If we try to stick her, we won't get anything anyway." As she spoke, her eyes were on the code room table. Dr. Newman was standing still with his hand inside the girl's chest, while the resident held the scalpel, widening the incision further.

"Listen," the chief blood-bank tech said, more calmly, almost pleading, "I don't need a lot. Just a little bit will be enough. I just can't keep sending un-cross-matched blood."

"You may have to," Heidi said. "They're opening her chest right now."

"Well for God's sake," the chief tech said plaintively, "isn't there blood gushing out somewhere that you can get me a little of?"

"Good point," Heidi said. "I'll get your blood for you." She hung up the phone, called instructions to a nurse, who, with a word to Newman, slipped a needleless syringe into the incision alongside his

165

gloved hand, and withdrew several cc of blood from inside the girl's chest cavity. She quickly capped the syringe, wrapped a label around it, and handed it to Heidi. As Heidi turned she almost bumped into Maggie, who was returning with a runner from the blood bank. Heidi handed the syringe to the runner. "Give this to your boss personally," she said.

◆ ◆ ◆

According to the chronological event sheet, Tanessa Starnes's heart began beating six minutes after she was wheeled into the code room. Some of the people who were there remember it as longer than that; a few say it was less. The truth is that time became meaningless in the headlong rush to save a child's life. Ordinarily, it takes fifteen minutes or so to open a chest, and that is with the proper instruments. Working with limited instruments and on sheer adrenaline, Kurt Newman had done it in less than five.

Now, with his left hand, he cradled Tanessa's heart, pressing gently with his thumb and middle finger on the two holes in her left ventricle. The pulse that he felt in his hand, and that showed now on the monitor screen, was extremely rapid, 150 beats per minute or more, as the heart raced to restore life to an oxygen-starved body. Tanessa's blood pressure began to rise, and as it did, the massive incision in her chest began to ooze dark blood.

"Clamp any major bleeders you can find," Newman instructed the surgical resident. "Let the rest go. We'll replace whatever volume she loses until we can get her into the OR."

His shoulder began to ache, and he shifted position slightly. He had to stand stooped over to keep his hand in place, and it was an awkward position. He couldn't stay that way indefinitely, but for the moment he couldn't move; with his fingers plugging the fatal bullet wound in the girl's heart, he literally held her life in his hand.

There was another worry as well. As any good surgeon must, Newman knew the anatomy of the human heart in intimate detail, and as his fingertips explored the surface of the pulsing muscle, his mind built up a three-dimensional picture of it. In his mental picture, the entrance wound was perilously close to one of the major vessels that supply blood to the heart itself. He brushed his forefinger along the heart's surface, feeling for the vein. If the bullet had severed that vein, then part of the heart's own blood supply was now being cut off by his finger, and the girl would be experiencing, for all intents and purposes, a heart attack. More correctly, it would be her second heart attack, the first being the heart failure caused by the bullet wound. And for the first time, the question intruded itself into Newman's mind: Can this girl survive?

"What do her pupils look like?" Newman asked the anesthesiologist at the head of the bed.

"None," the anesthesiologist replied. "Fixed and dilated."

Twice before in his medical career, Newman had treated children with similar wounds. Twice before, he had frantically torn open a child's chest right in the code room in a desperate struggle with death. Twice before he had lost. The odds were great that he would lose again. CPR is no substitute for a normal heartbeat; despite all their efforts, the girl could well be brain dead now, or worse, not quite dead but irreversibly brain damaged. Not to mention the incredible risk of infection: This was no ultrasterile operating suite; this was the code room, only a few feet from the bacteria-laden outdoors.

But the heart beat strongly inside Newman's hand. "Draw up some Kefzol, would you?" he said to the medications nurse. Kefzol is one of the new superpotent "miracle" antibiotics. As long as there was any faint shred of hope, Newman figured, the girl deserved the best they could give her.

◆ ◆ ◆

Dr. Frank Midgley, like Dr. Kurt Newman, was in the middle of a sterile surgical procedure when he was interrupted by the Tanessa Starnes case. Like Dr. Newman, Dr. Midgley immediately broke scrub, turned his case over to an assistant, and headed for the code room.

Dr. Newman had been answering Heidi's call for help; Dr. Midgley answered Dr. Newman's. Dr. Midgley is a specialist in pediatric cardiovascular surgery, with the intimate knowledge of children's circulatory systems that was suddenly required in the code room. As Dr. Newman had stood holding his hand around Tanessa's heart, he knew that he would quickly have to close the bullet holes in her left ventricle. For that he needed the help of a heart surgeon.

Kurt Newman is a general surgeon. As part of his training he has helped perform all different kinds of surgery, including heart and blood vessel surgery, and had there been no cardiovascular specialist in the hospital, he would have felt confident proceeding on his own. But heart surgery is a tricky and highly specialized business, more art than science. Tanessa's odds, whatever they were, would improve measurably with a heart surgeon in attendance. While a nurse held a telephone handset to Dr. Newman's ear, he conferred with Dr. Midgely, who was still in the second-floor surgical suite. Dr. Newman outlined the case in a few short sentences, and when Dr. Midgley arrived in the code room, he carried extra instruments and supplies for the repair job ahead.

It is no easy job to patch a hole in a beating heart. For one thing, the heart is moving all the time, which makes suturing difficult. For another thing, every time you remove your finger from the hole to try to plant a stitch, blood will come spurting out and hide all the important anatomic landmarks behind a red curtain. For yet another, the tissue of the heart is actually quite delicate, about the consistency of fine filet mignon. If mistreated, the heart muscle will tear, creating a series of problems that Tanessa clearly did not need.

The surgeons solved the problem with tiny plugs of sterile felt, called pledgets. The felt is absorbent enough to become filled with blood, but the blood, once there, forms a dense clot which closes off the bleeding. Dr. Newman removed a finger from the bullet wound in the front of Tanessa's heart, slapped a pledget over it, then held it in place with a fingertip while Dr. Midgley carefully attached it to the surface of the heart with a series of running sutures.

The back of the heart was tougher. The exit wound was larger, more ragged. Worse, they had to lift and turn the heart to be able to see the wound at all. If they lifted too high or turned too far, they might kink an important blood vessel, and Tanessa would fare poorly indeed. The two surgeons worked, bent over the teenager's body, carefully maneuvering the second pledget into place, then adding the sutures to hold it there.

Finally, the two men straightened. Newman flexed aching shoulder muscles. According to the chronological event sheet, only seventeen minutes had passed since he made his first incision in Tanessa's side. At the moment, it felt like an eternity.

Tanessa's heart, once the tamponade pressure had been released, had been beating strongly and with increasing steadiness. By a stroke of pure cosmic luck, the bullet had missed, by a millimeter, the artery that supplies the heart. As the two surgeons watched, the heart pulsed rhythmically, the sutures straining but holding at every heartbeat.

The job was far from finished; after exiting the heart, the bullet had torn holes in Tanessa's left lung. Those, too, would have to be repaired, but the immediate crisis was past; Tanessa's heart was beating, driving oxygen-rich blood through her body.

"I think it's safe to move her upstairs now," Newman said. Midgley nodded his agreement. "We can do our cleanup work there." At the word *cleanup,* he saw the resident's eyes dart across his midsection and downward. Stepping back from the table, he looked down and realized for the first time that his scrub suit pants were drenched in blood. His shoes made squishing noises as he shifted his weight from one foot to the other. He looked at the resident. "You're in charge," he said. "I'll see you in the OR in ten minutes." He strode off down the hall, toward the physicians' locker room, leaving a trail of jagged red footprints behind him.

Twenty-three _____

Anna Foster was a shy girl at a shy age, and try as they might, the nurses on 4-Blue never quite overcame that shyness. Anna was unfailingly polite; she stoically tolerated unpleasant and sometimes painful procedures that would have left other ten-year-olds in tears. Sometimes she even remembered to thank the nurses and technicians. But the rest of the time she was quiet and noticeably unchildish.

Indeed, Anna acted so grown-up that the nurses quietly arranged for a succession of people from social work and child life to drop in and visit with Anna and her mom and dad. The norm is for kids to cry; the nurses worry when they don't.

In Anna's case, they needn't have worried. Anna was perfectly normal—normal, that is, for a brilliant child. Anna, it turned out, was a straight-A student with an exceptionally high IQ and a voracious appetite for the printed word. Reading had broadened her outlook beyond her years. Not many ten-year-olds have the perspective to appreciate what hospitals do for them; Anna did.

But *appreciate* does not mean *enjoy*. Once she had been assured, first by her mother and then by several nurses and doctors, that she was not going to die, she concentrated all her energies on getting well enough to go home. She started breathing exercises even before the chest tube was out. When Mary Fallat told her that she'd heal faster if she walked around, she pulled on robe and slippers and paraded from one end of the hospital to the other as often as her exhausted parents would endure.

Between times, she grew more and more bored. She read Laura Ingalls Wilder books as fast as her parents could bring them in; when that wasn't enough, she borrowed a copy of the *Washington Post* from the 4-Blue nursing station and read that. Still she was bored, especially the last two days when the only impediment to her going home was a lingering low-grade fever. Dr. Fallat told Anna that drinking lots of water would help; Anna drank quarts of it. Sure enough the fever went down and stayed down. A week and a day after Nightmare Monday, Dr. Fallat announced that Anna could go home.

It was another brilliant spring day, and Anna sat in the back seat of the family car and sang songs during the ride home. She luxuriated in the sunshine, gaped at the unfamiliar scenery of downtown Washington, and cried real tears when she found out she couldn't go back to school the next morning. By the time she got home, though, she was exhausted and agreed reluctantly that she needed more rest before she could go back to school.

Her brother Larry had been just as happy when he got to go home the Friday before—that is, until he got a visit from Cyndy Wright, who had forbidden him to ride a bicycle, roller skate, play football, or do anything else that might reinjure his healing spleen. Then, having outlawed all the fun things, Cyndy said it would be perfectly okay for Larry to go back to school the following Monday. Larry was a bit young to use words like *injustice,* but the look on his face clearly conveyed the sentiment.

◆ ◆ ◆

Tanessa Starnes walked gingerly, as though her feet hurt, and she held one arm against the front of her torso, where her healing surgical wounds were still sore, but she smiled brightly as the cameras flashed away, and when she stepped up to a bank of microphones her first words, soft but clear, were "Hi. I feel fine."

It was a low-key performance. It became spectacular only when you remembered that this was the girl who, ten days before, had entered the code room with no pulse or blood pressure, and who had been literally torn open on the code room examining table so that Kurt Newman could use his fingers to plug the bullet holes in her heart.

Now Dr. Newman and Tanessa's father, a pair of Tanessa's nurses, along with Marion Barry, the mayor of Washington, D.C., and paramedics Donna Beverly, Van Coppedge, and John Proper, all stood around Tanessa the Miracle Girl and smiled while the photographers and cameramen had a field day.

The truth, Kurt Newman said later, is that there were no miracles, just a great deal of luck. Tanessa was lucky that the first ambulance to reach her contained well-trained and aggressive medics who refused to give up on her, even when her heartbeat and breathing had stopped.

But most of all, she was lucky that she lived in Washington, D.C., near the Children's Hospital National Medical Center, where back in 1980 Marty Eichelberger started a pediatric trauma service. You might say that Marty's trauma people had been rehearsing their ballet for seven years to get ready for Tanessa's arrival.

"It's wonderful to have a system," Newman says. "Everything's already in place; all you have to do is call for it. All I had to do was look at people, say half a word, and it was done. All the pieces were already there, and one by one they fell right into place."

That was after the fact, though: The night Kurt Newman sewed up Tanessa's punctured heart, the adrenaline kept him wide awake until the small hours of the morning, but he fell asleep believing that there wouldn't be a lot left of the life he had saved. The "insult," as doctors call it, had simply been too great for any fourteen-year-old girl to endure.

He began to have second thoughts the next morning, when he made rounds and the nurses told him she had begun to move her arms and legs. He made rounds again at midday, and learned that she had begun to thrash about in bed. He came back to the ICU twice during the afternoon and was as shocked and thrilled as everyone else when Tanessa opened her eyes and looked around.

Even now, when Newman sits in his office and talks about it, he occasionally shakes his head as though still not quite ready to believe it. "It was perfect," he says. "Perfect. Everything happened just like it was supposed to. We did all the right things; we got all the breaks." There are medical and anatomic reasons why things worked out so well, and Newman explains them in the precise language of a surgeon, but then his words drift off, and again he shakes his head. "It was the sort of thing," he says, "that if you're lucky happens to you once in an entire career."

Or, if you're Tanessa Starnes, once in a lifetime.

◆ ◆ ◆

Little David Myers, in his own way, beat all the odds, too. By all rights he should have died on Alabama Avenue, within sight of his home, but the child had a toughness, a sort of natural resilience, about him that everyone underestimated from the beginning. By all rights he should have died in the hospital during the critical twenty-four hours after the accident, but that toughness, and the constant attention of the residents and the nurses, brought him through the crisis period alive.

When little David didn't wake up on schedule, his physicians got gloomy again. They were only being realistic, figuring the averages, but Children's Hospital is not always a place where the averages apply.

The doctors had said his vocal cords were ruined and that he would never speak; yet by the time he left for the Kennedy Institute, he had learned to hold a finger over his tracheostomy tube so he could gather up the windpower to say "Hi."

The doctors had said his brain was so badly damaged that he would never see. His eyes were fine, they said, but the part of his brain that processed images was gone. Cortical blindness, they called it. The worst kind. The kind that never gets better. But then, one weekend at the Ronald McDonald House across from the Kennedy Institute, Mr. Myers discovered that if he stood to David's right, the boy smiled. If he moved to the left, the smile vanished. The following Monday, the therapists at Kennedy tested David's vision and sure enough, he had regained partial sight, enough to get around.

By the time Mr. Myers brought David back to Children's Hospital for his six-month checkup, the boy was walking, playing with toys, and fitting words together into simple sentences. Even Dr. Laura Tosi, the feisty, hard-boiled orthopedic surgeon who had supervised the repair of David's legs, fairly bubbled with delight.

"He has done about a thousand percent better than any of us dreamed he would," Dr. Tosi told Mr. Myers, while David wheeled a toy truck around the examining room floor and occasionally up the walls.

Dr. Tosi was one of the many pessimists on the team of physicians who took care of little David. Despite her crusty exterior, Dr. Tosi, like everyone else at Children's Hospital, loves kids and loves happy endings. She snapped fresh X-rays onto a lightbox and pointed with a pencil. "His legs have healed much better than we expected them to," she told Mr. Myers. "You can see here," she said, pointing, "how the bones have aligned themselves very nicely, and now the callus— the excess bone around the fracture site—has already begun to dissolve away. In a few years, you won't be able to tell the leg was ever broken."

Little David, thoroughly bored with the proceedings, sent the truck sailing across the floor and crashed it, with a satisfying racket, into a stainless steel trash can. Mr. Myers jumped, then shook an angry finger at his son. "David! Don't do that!" he said sharply.

David turned his head, slowly, until he could see his father. An impish grin spread across his face. "Okay," he said, as he reached for the truck.

Postscript ———————————
A CALL TO ARMS

There is a chance that you, the reader, having finished this tale of what Marty Eichelberger has done in Washington, D.C., may now wonder, on behalf of your own children or your neighbor's, what sort of pediatric trauma services are available near you. Chances are there are none, but that does not mean there is nothing you can do. You can be prepared. The secret of trauma care is in the preparation.

Obviously, your first and most important relationship is with your family pediatrician. But if there are pediatric surgeons in your town, it would be a good idea to know their names. Serious injuries often require surgical repair, and simply knowing the right names can save precious time.

On a family level, planning is important. Just as every family should have a fire plan, every family should have an accident plan. Children should learn the local emergency phone number as soon as they learn to dial the phone; parents can consult with the family pediatrician for the names of the best-equipped hospitals, best-qualified surgeons, and so on. The main point is to have a plan in advance so that if, God forbid, something does happen, you won't have to improvise on the spot; you'll know, step by step, what you have to do.

While thinking the unthinkable, take time to review your medical insurance. In the last few years, the struggle to reduce medical costs has produced many budget-conscious enterprises such as "preferred provider" plans and health maintenance organizations. Preferred provider insurance could require you to take an injured child only to certain hospitals. Make sure that one of those hospitals has adequate facilities to care for injured children. Likewise, if you belong to an HMO, it would be a good idea to examine your contract closely to see what limitations the HMO places on such things as rehabilitation and restorative therapy. Seriously injured children often require a great deal of rehab work to recover fully, and many HMOs will balk at the expense. Depending on the type of insurance coverage you have, you may want to consider supplementary "catastrophic" insurance coverage.

Above all, practice accident prevention. Try to imagine all the myriad ways in which a child can get hurt, and take preventive measures. There are no guarantees, of course, but with a few precautions you can improve the odds dramatically.

There is another level of concern at which parents can become active, and that is the community, or the political level. Good trauma care, for both adults and children, depends on several things.

First, there must be good prehospital care. The ambulance medics who answer the call must have adequate equipment and adequate training. Lacking either the proper hardware or the proper knowledge, a well-meaning medic can do an injured child as much harm as good.

All states, by law, have emergency medical services programs, and those EMS programs, among other things, are responsible for training paramedics. There are state and national standards for what sort of training paramedics ought to have and how often they should receive refresher courses. State EMS offices know what those standards are, and they also know how closely the ambulance services under their jurisdiction adhere to the standards. The information is there; if you are willing to take on your state bureaucracy, you can find out, in great detail, just how good your local ambulance service really is, compared to how good it could be. At the end of this chapter you will find a list of the fifty state EMS directors. By now some of the names will surely have changed, but the offices will not. To begin learning about pediatric emergency care in your state, the EMS director's office is the best starting point.

Second, your local hospital, no matter how large or small, ought to have the basic equipment needed to treat pediatric emergencies. What does that mean? It means the hospital's emergency room ought to have, on hand and immediately available, a full collection of pediatric supplies: airway tubes in all sizes, chest tubes in all sizes, IV sets in all sizes, Foley catheters in all sizes. You can't use adult-size supplies on a two-year-old; without the proper tools, even the best physician can do little good. All hospitals have boards of directors or other governing bodies; if your local hospital doesn't measure up, take it up with the board.

Your local hospital ought to have a CAT scanner. This one diagnostic device has saved hundreds of injured children from exploratory surgery. Most hospitals have the scanners; if yours doesn't, then perhaps it is time for a community fund drive.

Third, there must be a communications system. Not every hospital can afford to have pediatric trauma specialists available around the clock, but the very large ones can, and they have telephones. If a small hospital has the proper equipment on hand, and its physicians can get expert advice instantly by phone, your child's chances improve dramatically.

Fourth, your state or your region must have a hierarchy of hospitals. All hospitals ought to be equipped to treat minor trauma; at least one hospital in each region ought to be capable of handling serious and possibly life-threatening injury. And at central points throughout the country, there should be highly sophisticated trauma centers, staffed and equipped to deal with multiple life-threatening injuries. Most major metropolitan areas have such trauma centers for adults; very few have comparable centers for children.

There is no excuse for this, politically or economically. The trauma center has been a financial success at Children's Hospital National Medical Center, and similar centers could be equally successful in other major cities. Any city with a medical school or a teaching hospital has a pediatrics program, including at least some facilities for pediatric surgery. If that hospital can meet certain standards, it can be designated as a pediatric trauma center, and the paramedics in the field will be told to deliver injured children directly there, bypassing other hospitals. As the hospital staff acquire more and more experience treating injured kids, they will do a better and better job of it. Meanwhile, the hospital will benefit financially from the steady stream of high-revenue patients, many of whom are heavily insured.

Fifth, there must be a statewide radio communications system to coordinate the efforts of the medics in the field and the doctors and nurses in the emergency room. Without a communications system, Tanessa Starnes would have shown up unannounced at the Children's emergency room door, and precious minutes would have been wasted in organizing the trauma team. Tanessa lives because in Washington there is an organized, systematic approach to trauma care, and communications is a vital part of that system.

Sixth, there must be air transport available. Not every city can have its own children's trauma center, but every city should have timely access to one. Many states have flying ambulances, med-evac helicopters available round the clock. In more remote areas, fixed-wing craft can substitute. Most areas of the country now have some sort of air-ambulance service. The nearest children's trauma center should be less than an hour away by whatever means of transportation is available.

✦ ✦ ✦

Those are the components of every successful trauma system. State government, usually the health department, coordinates all these things. When one or more components are missing, lives may be lost. Happily, trauma is one of the few problems that can always be solved by throwing money at it. Where something is lacking, money will fix it.

✦ ✦ ✦

To assist you in establishing or refining the emergency care system that serves your children and your community, I have compiled three lists. The first is a listing of pediatric hospitals, their addresses, and the relevant services they provide. The list is undoubtedly incomplete; I have probably overlooked some children's hospitals, and I have made no attempt to include all hospitals that have pediatric services. This list includes only the exclusively pediatric hospitals. It is a starting point, and only that: a list of resources where, if nothing else, you can call or write for more information.

The principal national resource, the one this book was about, is Children's Hospital National Medical Center, and inquiries can be sent directly to them:

Trauma Service
Children's Hospital National Medical Center
111 Michigan Avenue, N.W.
Washington, D.C.   20010

The next list contains the names of EMS directors in the United States and territories. By now some of the names are likely to have changed, but the offices probably have not, and the state EMS program is always a good starting point, whether your goal is a free-standing children's trauma center in your community or simply better-trained paramedics.

The final list contains the names of graduates of the pediatric EMS training program that was described briefly in the book. These people are instructors, people who teach paramedics how to be paramedics. They have all been through the week-long, total-immersion course at Children's Hospital; they know all about the special needs of injured children, and they know how to teach that information to others. If the paramedics in your community haven't received pediatric training, these are the people to contact.

◆ ◆ ◆

Eight thousand children die in accidents every year. Fifty thousand more are disabled. Many of those accidents could be prevented, and where prevention fails, many more lives could be saved with proper trauma care. We can, and must, do something.

Appendix I ─────────
PEDIATRIC HOSPITALS:

UNITED STATES

ALABAMA

Children's Hospital of Alabama
1600 Sixth Avenue, South
Birmingham, AL 35233
(205) 939–9100
160 Beds
Intensive Care Unit
Emergency Room

U. of S. Alabama Medical Center
Children and Women's Hospital
2451 Fillingim Street
Mobile, AL 36617
(205) 471–7506
Emergency Room
Intensive Care Unit

ARKANSAS

Arkansas Children's Hospital
804 Wolfe Street
Little Rock, AR 72202
(501) 370–1100
176 Beds
Intensive Care Unit

Outpatient Rehabilitation
Emergency Room

CALIFORNIA

Children's Hospital and Health Center
8001 Frost Street
San Diego, CA 92123
(619) 576–1700
Intensive Care Unit
Outpatient Rehabilitation

Children's Hospital of Los Angeles
4650 Sunset Boulevard
Box 54700
Los Angeles, CA 90054
(213) 660–2450
317 Beds
Intensive Care Unit
Outpatient Rehabilitation
Emergency Room
Inpatient Rehabilitation

Children's Hospital Medical Center of Northern California

51st and Grove Streets
Oakland, CA 94609
(415) 428–3000
142 Beds
Intensive Care Unit
Outpatient Rehabilitation
Emergency Room

Children's Hospital of Orange
County
1109 West LaVeta Avenue
Orange, CA 92668
(714) 997–3000
151 Beds
Intensive Care Unit

Children's Hospital at Stanford
520 Willow Road
Palo Alto, CA 94304
(415) 327–4800
60 Beds
Intensive Care Unit
Outpatient Rehabilitation

Devereux Foundation
Box 1079
Santa Barbara, CA 93102
(805) 968–2525
190 Beds

Shriners Hospitals For Crippled Children
3160 Geneva Street
Los Angeles, CA 90020
(213) 388–3151
60 Beds
Intensive Care Unit
Outpatient Rehabilitation

Shriners Hospitals For Crippled Children
1701 19th Avenue
San Francisco, CA 94122
(415) 665–1100
50 Beds
Intensive Care Unit

Southwood Psychiatric Hospital
950 Third Avenue
Chula Vista, CA 92011
(619) 426–6310
88 Beds

Valley Children's Hospital
3151 North Millbrook Avenue
Fresno, CA 93703
(209) 225–3000
112 Beds
Intensive Care Unit
Emergency Room

COLORADO

Children's Hospital
1056 East 19th Avenue
Denver, CO 80218
(303) 861–8888
173 Beds
Intensive Care Unit
Outpatient Rehabilitation
Emergency Room

CONNECTICUT

Housatonic Adolescent Hospital
Box W

Newtown, CT 06470
(203) 426–2531
35 Beds

Newington Children's Hospital
181 East Cedar Street
Newington, CT 06111
(203) 667–5437
98 Beds
Intensive Care Unit
Inpatient Rehabilitation
Outpatient Rehabilitation

Riverview Hospital For
Children
River Road, Box 621
Middletown, CT 06457
(203) 344–2700
57 Beds

DELAWARE

Alfred I. DuPont Institute
P.O. Box 269
Wilmington, DE 19899
(302) 651–4000
60 Beds
Intensive Care Unit
Inpatient Rehabilitation
Outpatient Rehabilitation

DISTRICT OF COLOMBIA

Children's Hospital National
Medical Center
111 Michigan Avenue, N.W.
Washington, DC 20010
(202) 745–5188
263 Beds

Intensive Care Unit
Outpatient Rehabilitation
Trauma Center

Hospital For Sick Children
1731 Bunker Hill Road, N.E.
Washington, DC 20017
(202) 832–4400
80 Beds
Outpatient Rehabilitation
Inpatient Rehabilitation

FLORIDA

All Children's Hospital
801 Sixth Street, South
St. Petersburg, FL 33701
(813) 898–7451
80 Beds
Intensive Care Unit
Inpatient Rehabilitation
Outpatient Rehabilitation
Emergency Room

Grant Center Hospital
Box 1159
Miami, FL 33197
(305) 251–0710
100 Beds

The Miami Children's Hospital
6125 S.W. 31st Street
Miami, FL 33155
(305) 666–6511
188 Beds
Intensive Care Unit
Outpatient Rehabilitation
Emergency Room

Nemours Children's Hospital
5720 Atlantic Boulevard
Jacksonville, FL 32207
(904) 725–1600

GEORGIA

Anneewakee Hospital
4771 Anneewakee Road
Douglasville, GA 30135
(404) 942–2391
315 Beds

Devereux Center
1980 Stanley Road
Kennesaw, GA 30144
(404) 427–0147
77 Beds

Henrietta Egleston Hospital
For Children
1405 Clifton Road, N.E.
Atlanta, GA 30322
(404) 325–6000
142 Beds
Intensive Care Unit

Scottish Rite Children's Hospital
1001 Johnson Ferry Road, N.E.
Atlanta, GA 30363
(404) 256–5252
76 Beds
Intensive Care Unit
Emergency Room

HAWAII

Kapiolani—Children's Medical
Center

1319 Punahou Street
Honolulu, HI 96826
(808) 947–8511
70 Beds
Intensive Care Unit
Outpatient Rehabilitation
Emergency Room

Shriners Hospitals For Crippled Children
1310 Punahou Street
Honolulu, HI 96826
(808) 941–4466
40 Beds
Intensive Care Unit
Outpatient Rehabilitation

ILLINOIS

Children's Memorial Hospital
2300 Children's Plaza
Chicago, IL 60614
(312) 880–4000
250 Beds
Intensive Care Unit
Emergency Room

Larabida Children's Hospital
and Research Center
East 65th Street at Lake Michigan
Chicago, IL 60649
(312) 363–6700
77 Beds
Intensive Care Unit
Outpatient Rehabilitation
Emergency Room

Shriners Hospitals For Crippled Children

2211 North Oak Park Avenue
Chicago, IL 60635
(312) 622–5400
60 Beds
Intensive Care Unit
Outpatient Rehabilitation

KANSAS

Children's Division of Menninger Foundation
P.O. Box 829
Topeka, KS 66601
(913) 273–7500
68 Beds

KENTUCKY

Kosair—Children's Hospital of NKC, Inc.
P.O. Box 35070
Louisville, KY 40232
(502) 562–6000
277 Beds
Intensive Care Unit
Emergency Room

Shriners Hospitals For Crippled Children
1900 Richmond Road
Lexington, KY 40502
(606) 266–2101
50 Beds
Intensive Care Unit
Outpatient Rehabilitation

LOUISIANA

Children's Hospital
200 Henry Clay Avenue

New Orleans, LA 70118
(504) 899–9511
91 Beds
Intensive Care Unit
Inpatient Rehabilitation
Outpatient Rehabilitation
Emergency Room

Shriners Hospitals For Crippled Children
3100 Samford Avenue
Shreveport, LA 71103
(318) 222–5704
30 Beds
Intensive Care Unit
Outpatient Rehabilitation

MARYLAND

Johns Hopkins Hospital
600 North Wolfe Street
Baltimore, MD 21205
(301) 955–5000
Emergency Room
Intensive Care Unit

John F. Kennedy Institute
707 North Broadway
Baltimore, MD 21205
(301) 522–5407
40 Beds
Inpatient Rehabilitation
Outpatient Rehabilitation

Mt. Washington Pediatric Hospital
1708 West Rogers Avenue
Baltimore, MD 21209
(301) 578–8600

62 Beds
Outpatient Rehabilitation
Inpatient Rehabilitation

MASSACHUSETTS

Children's Hospital
300 Longwood Avenue
Boston, MA 02115
(617) 735–6000
339 Beds
Intensive Care Unit
Outpatient Rehabilitation
Emergency Room

Joseph P. Kennedy, Jr., Memorial Hospital
30 Warren Street, Brighton
Boston, MA 02135
(617) 254–3800
100 Beds
Inpatient Rehabilitation
Outpatient Rehabilitation
Emergency Room

Shriners Burns Institute
51 Blossom Street
Boston, MA 02114
(617) 722–3000
30 Beds

Floating Hospital For Infants &
Children
171 Harrison Avenue
Boston, MA 02111
(617) 956–5000
102 Beds
Intensive Care Unit
Emergency Room

Massachusetts Hospital School
3 Randolph Street
Canton, MA 02021
(617) 828–2440
Intensive Care Unit
Outpatient Rehabilitation

North Shore Children's Hospital
57 Highland Avenue
Salem, MA 01970
(617) 745–2100
50 Beds
Intensive Care Unit
Emergency Room

Shriners Hospitals For Crippled Children
516 Carew Street
Springfield, MA 01104
(413) 781–6750
60 Beds
Intensive Care Unit
Outpatient Rehabilitation

MICHIGAN

Children's Hospital of Michigan
3901 Beaubien Boulevard
Detroit, MI 48201
(313) 494–5301
282 Beds
Intensive Care Unit
Outpatient Rehabilitation
Emergency Room

Hawthorn Center
18471 Haggerty Road

Northville, MI 48167
(313) 349–3000
136 Beds
Intensive Care Unit

MINNESOTA

Children's Hospital
345 North Smith Avenue
St. Paul, MN 55102
(612) 298–8666
98 Beds
Intensive Care Unit
Emergency Room

Gillette Children's Hospital
200 East University Avenue
St. Paul, MN 55101
(612) 291–2848
54 Beds
Intensive Care Unit
Outpatient Rehabilitation

Minneapolis Children's Medical Center
2525 Chicago Avenue, South
Minneapolis, MN 55404
(612) 874–6100
107 Beds
Intensive Care Unit
Emergency Room

Shriners Hospitals For Crippled Children
2025 East River Road
Minneapolis, MN 55414
(612) 339–6711
40 Beds
Intensive Care Unit
Outpatient Rehabilitation

MISSOURI

Cardinal Glennon Memorial
Hospital
1465 South Grand Boulevard
St. Louis, MO 63104
(314) 577–5600
190 Beds
Intensive Care Unit
Emergency Room

Children's Mercy Hospital
24th at Gillham Road
Kansas City, MO 64108
(816) 234–3000
151 Beds
Intensive Care Unit
Outpatient Rehabilitation
Emergency Room

Crittenton Center
10918 Elm Avenue
Kansas City, MO 64134
(816) 765–6600
67 Beds

H.S.A. Heartland Hospital
Ashland & Prewitt Streets
Nevada, MO 64772
(417) 667–2666
100 Beds
Inpatient Rehabilitation

St. Louis Children's Hospital
400 South Kingshighway Boulevard
Box 14871
St. Louis, MO 63178
(314) 454–6000

182 Beds
Intensive Care Unit
Emergency Room

Shriners Hospitals For Crippled Children
2001 South Lindbergh Boulevard
St. Louis, MO 63131
(314) 432–3600
80 Beds
Intensive Care Unit
Outpatient Rehabilitation

Weldon Spring Hospital
5931 Highway 94 South
St. Charles, MO 63301
(314) 441–7300
72 Beds

MONTANA

Shodair Children's Hospital
840 Helena Avenue
Helena, MT 59604
(406) 442–1980
31 Beds
Emergency Room

NEBRASKA

Boys Town Institute For Communications Disorders in Children
555 North 30th Street
Omaha, NE 68131
(402) 449–6511
42 Beds

Children's Memorial Hospital
8301 Dodge Street
Omaha, NE 68114
(402) 390–5450
100 Beds
Intensive Care Unit
Emergency Room

NEW JERSEY

Children's Hospital of New Jersey of
United Hospitals Medical Center
15 South Ninth Street
Newark, NJ 07107
(201) 268–8760
122 Beds
Intensive Care Unit

Children's Seashore House
4100 Atlantic Avenue
Atlantic City, NJ 08404
(609) 345–5191
64 Beds
Inpatient Rehabilitation
Outpatient Rehabilitation

Children's Specialized Hospital
New Providence Road
Mountainside, NJ 07091
(201) 233–3720
60 Beds
Outpatient Rehabilitation

Matheny School
Main Street
Peapack, NJ 07977

(201) 234–0011
Inpatient Rehabilitation

NEW MEXICO

Carrie Tingley Crippled Children's Hospital
P.O. Box 25447
Albuquerque, NM 87125
(505) 841–9121
27 Beds
Intensive Care Unit
Inpatient Rehabilitation
Outpatient Rehabilitation

NEW YORK

Blythedale Children's Hospital
Bradhurst Avenue
Valhalla, NY 10595
(914) 592–7555
92 Beds
Intensive Care Unit
Outpatient Rehabilitation
Inpatient Rehabilitation

Bronx Children's Psychiatric
Center
1000 Waters Place
New York, NY 10461
(212) 892–0808
75 Beds
Intensive Care Unit
Outpatient Rehabilitation

Children's Hospital of Buffalo
219 Bryant Street
Buffalo, NY 14222
(716) 878–7000

246 Beds
Intensive Care Unit
Outpatient Rehabilitation
Emergency Room

Queens Children's Psychiatric
Center
74-03 Commonwealth Boulevard
New York, NY 11426
(212) 464–2900
173 Beds

Rockland Children's Psychiatric Center
Convent Road
Orangeburg, NY 10962
(914) 359–7400
104 Beds

Sagamore Children's Center
Half Hollow Road
Melville, NY 11747
(516) 673–7700
122 Beds

Western New York Child's
Psychiatric Center
1010 East and West Road
West Seneca, NY 14224
(716) 674–9730
60 Beds

NORTH CAROLINA

Lenox Baker Children's Hospital
3000 Erwin Road
Durham, NC 27705

189

(919) 683–6890
40 Beds
Outpatient Rehabilitation

OHIO

Children's Hospital
700 Children's Drive
Columbus, OH 43205
(614) 461–2000
313 Beds
Intensive Care Unit
Emergency Room

Children's Hospital Medical
Center
Elland and Bethesda Avenues
Cincinnati, OH 45229
(513) 559–4200
350 Beds
Intensive Care Unit
Outpatient Rehabilitation
Emergency Room

Children's Hospital Medical
Center of Akron
281 Locust Street
Akron, OH 44308
(216) 379–8200
253 Beds
Intensive Care Unit
Outpatient Rehabilitation
Emergency Room

Children's Medical Center
One Children's Plaza
Dayton, OH 45404
(513) 226–8300
152 Beds

Intensive Care Unit
Outpatient Rehabilitation
Emergency Room

Health Hill Hospital For Children
2801 Martin Luther King, Jr.,
Drive
Cleveland, OH 44104
(216) 721–5400
52 Beds
Outpatient Rehabilitation
Inpatient Rehabilitation

Sagamore Hills Children's Psychiatric Hospital
11910 Dunham Road
Northfield, OH 44067
(216) 467–7955
64 Beds

Shriners Hospitals For Crippled Children,
Shriners Burns Institute
Cincinnati Unit
202 Goodman Street
Cincinnati, OH 45219
(513) 751–3900
30 Beds

Tod Babies' & Children's Hospital
500 Gypsy Lane
Youngstown, OH 44501
(216) 747–1444
95 Beds
Intensive Care Unit

OKLAHOMA

Children's Medical Center
5300 East Skelly Drive
Box 35648
Tulsa, OK 74135
(918) 664–6600
101 Beds
Intensive Care Unit
Outpatient Rehabilitation

Shadow Mountain Institute
6262 South Sheridan
Tulsa, OK 74133
(918) 492–8200
135 Beds
Intensive Care Unit

OREGON

Shriners Hospitals For Crippled Children
3101 S.W. Sam Jackson Park Road
Portland, OR 97201
(503) 241–5090
40 Beds
Intensive Care Unit
Outpatient Rehabilitation

PENNSYLVANIA

Children's Heart Hospital
Conshohocken Avenue
Philadelphia, PA 19131
(215) 877–7708
65 Beds
Outpatient Rehabilitation

Children's Hospital of Philadelphia
34th Street & Civic Center Boulevard
Philadelphia, PA 19104
(215) 596–9100
245 Beds
Intensive Care Unit
Outpatient Rehabilitation
Emergency Room

Children's Hospital of Pittsburgh
125 DeSoto Street
Pittsburgh, PA 15213
(412) 647–5010
230 Beds
Intensive Care Unit
Outpatient Rehabilitation
Emergency Room

Eastern State School and Hospital
3740 Lincoln Highway
Trevose, PA 19047
(215) 671–3141
182 Beds

Rehabilitation Institute of Pittsburgh
6301 Northumberland Street
Pittsburgh, PA 15217
(412) 521–9000
124 Beds
Outpatient Rehabilitation
Inpatient Rehabilitation

St. Christopher's Hospital For Children

191

5th Street & Lehigh Avenue
Philadelphia, PA 19133
(215) 427–5000
146 Beds
Intensive Care Unit
Outpatient Rehabilitation
Emergency Room

Shriners Hospitals For Crippled Children
1645 West Eighth Street
Erie, PA 16505
(814) 456–7565
30 Beds
Intensive Care Unit
Outpatient Rehabilitation

Shriners Hospitals For Crippled Children
8400 Roosevelt Boulevard
Philadelphia, PA 19152
(215) 332–4500
80 Beds
Intensive Care Unit
Inpatient Rehabilitation
Outpatient Rehabilitation

D. T. Watson Rehabilitation
Hospital
Camp Meeting Road
Sewickley, PA 15143
(412) 741–9500
50 Beds
Outpatient Rehabilitation

RHODE ISLAND

Emma Pendleton Bradley Hospital

1011 Veterans Memorial Parkway
Riverside, RI 02915
(401) 434–3400
56 Beds
Intensive Care Unit

SOUTH CAROLINA

Shriners Hospitals For Crippled Children
2100 North Pleasantburg Drive
Greenville, SC 29609
(803) 244–4530
62 Beds
Intensive Care Unit
Outpatient Rehabilitation

SOUTH DAKOTA

Crippled Children's Hospital &
School
2501 West 26th Street
Sioux Falls, SD 57105
(605) 336–1840
92 Beds
Outpatient Rehabilitation

TENNESSEE

East Tennessee Children's Hospital
2018 Clinch Avenue
Knoxville, TN 37916
(615) 546–7711
100 Beds
Intensive Care Unit
Emergency Room

Le Bonheur Children's Medical
Center
One Children's Plaza
Memphis, TN 38103
(901) 522–3000
152 Beds
Intensive Care Unit
Outpatient Rehabilitation
Emergency Room

Metropolitan Hospital
511 McCallie Avenue
Chattanooga, TN 37402
(615) 265–3303
64 Beds
Emergency Room

St. Jude Children's Research
Hospital
332 North Lauderdale Street
Memphis, TN 38101
(901) 522–0300
48 Beds
Intensive Care Unit

TEXAS

Children's Medical Center of
Dallas
1935 Amelia Street
Dallas, TX 75235
(214) 920–2000
158 Beds
Intensive Care Unit

W. T. Cook Children's Hospital
1212 West Lancaster Street
Fort Worth, TX 76102

(817) 336–5521
67 Beds
Emergency Room

Devereux Foundation
Box 2666
Victoria, TX 77901
(512) 575–8271
165 Beds

Driscoll Foundation Children's
Hospital
3533 South Alameda Street
Drawer 6530
Corpus Christi, TX 78411
(512) 854–5341
132 Beds
Intensive Care Unit
Emergency Room

Fort Worth Children's Hospital
1400 Cooper Street
Fort Worth, TX 76104
(817) 336–9861
88 Beds
Intensive Care Unit

Methodist Home Children's
Guidance Center
1111 Herring Avenue
Waco, TX 76708
(817) 753–0181
20 Beds

Oaks Treatment Center—
Brown Schools
1407 Stassney Lane
Austin, TX 78745
(512) 444–9561

193

120 Beds
Intensive Care Unit

San Antonio Children's Center
2939 West Woodlawn
San Antonio, TX 78228
(512) 736–4273
60 Beds
Intensive Care Unit

Shriners Hospitals For Crip-
pled Children,
Burns Institute
Galveston Unit
610 Texas Avenue
Galveston, TX 77550
(409) 761–2516
30 Beds
Intensive Care Unit
Outpatient Rehabilitation

Shriners Hospitals For Crippled Children
1402 Outer Belt Drive
Houston, TX 77030
(713) 797–1616
40 Beds
Intensive Care Unit
Outpatient Rehabilitation

Texas Children's Hospital
P.O. Box 20269
Houston, TX 77225
(713) 791–2070
307 Beds
Intensive Care Unit
Outpatient Rehabilitation
Emergency Room

Texas Scottish Rite Hospital
For Crippled Children
2222 Welborn Street
Box 19567
Dallas, TX 75219
(214) 521–3168
64 Beds
Intensive Care Unit
Outpatient Rehabilitation

UTAH

Primary Children's Hospital
320 12th Avenue
Salt Lake City, UT 84103
(801) 363–1221
164 Beds
Intensive Care Unit
Inpatient Rehabilitation
Outpatient Rehabilitation
Emergency Room

Shriners Hospitals For Crip-
pled Children
Fairfax Avenue & Virginia
Street
Salt Lake City, UT 84103
(801) 532–5307
45 Beds
Intensive Care Unit

VIRGINIA

Charter Colonial Institute
17579 Warwick Boulevard
Newport News, VA 23603
(804) 887–2611
60 Beds

Children's Hospital, Inc.
2924 Brook Road
Richmond, VA 23220
(804) 321–7474
30 Beds
Intensive Care Unit
Outpatient Rehabilitation

Children's Hospital of the King's Daughters
800 West Olney Road
Norfolk, VA 23507
(804) 628–3740
128 Beds
Intensive Care Unit

Children's Rehabilitation Center
University of Virginia Hospital
2270 Ivy Road
Charlottesville, VA 22901
(804) 924–5500
39 Beds
Intensive Care Unit
Inpatient Rehabilitation
Outpatient Rehabilitation
Emergency Room

De Jarnette Center
Richmond Road, Box 2309
Staunton, VA 24401
(703) 885–9050
60 Beds

Graydon Manor
301 Children's Center Road
Leesburg, VA 22075
(703) 777–3485
61 Beds

Psychiatric Institute of Richmond
3001 Fifth Avenue
Richmond, VA 23222
(804) 329–4392
84 Beds
Intensive Care Unit
Outpatient Rehabilitation

WASHINGTON

Children's Orthopedic Hospital
4800 Sand Point Way N.E.
Box C-5371
Seattle, WA 98105
(206) 526–2000
197 Beds
Intensive Care Unit
Inpatient Rehabilitation
Outpatient Rehabilitation
Emergency Room

Mary Bridge Children's Health Center
311 South L Street, Box 5588
Tacoma, WA 98405
(206) 594–1400
82 Beds
Intensive Care Unit
Outpatient Rehabilitation
Emergency Room

Shriners Hospitals For Crippled Children
North 820 Summit Boulevard
Spokane, WA 99201
(509) 327–9521
30 Beds
Intensive Care Unit

WISCONSIN

Milwaukee Children's Hospital
1700 West Wisconsin Avenue
Milwaukee, WI 53233

(414) 931–1010
170 Beds
Intensive Care Unit
Outpatient Rehabilitation
Emergency Room

Appendix II _____
STATE EMS DIRECTORS

ALABAMA

Arthur Harman
Director, Department of
Health, EMS
State Office Building
Room 644
Montgomery, AL 36130–1701
(205) 832–3935

ALASKA

Mark Johnson
Coordinator, EMS
Department of Health & Social
Service
Pouch H-06C
Juneau, AK 99811
(602) 220–6400

ARIZONA

Irene Conlan
Assistant Director
EMS & Health Care Facilities
Arizona Department of Health
Services
411 North 24th Street

Phoenix, AZ 85008
(602) 220–6400

ARKANSAS

Michael L. Hampton
Director, Office of EMS
Department of Health
4815 West Markham Street
Little Rock, AR 72201
(501) 661–2262

CALIFORNIA

Bruce E. Haynes, M.D.
Director, EMS Authority
1030 15th Street, Suite 302
Sacramento, CA 95814
(916) 322–4336

COLORADO

William Metcalf
Director, EMS Division
Department of Health
4210 East 11th Avenue
Denver, CO 80220
(303) 320–8333

Alan Doelp

CONNECTICUT

Mr. Chris A. Gentile
Director, Office of EMS
Department of Health
150 Washington Street
Hartford, CT 06106
(203) 566–4445

DELAWARE

Charles E. Nabb
Director of EMS
Capitol Square
Jesse S. Cooper Memorial
Building
Dover, DE 19901
(302) 736–4710

DISTRICT OF COLOMBIA

Mary Berkeley
Chief
Emergency Health & Medical
Services
1875 Connecticut Avenue, N.W.
Room 833D
Washington, DC 20009
(202) 673–6744

FLORIDA

Larry S. Jordan
Administrator, EMS
Department of Health & Reha-
bilitation
1317 Winewood Building #8
Room 110

Tallahassee, FL 32301
(904) 487–1911

GEORGIA

Mrs. Dallas Jankowski, J.D.
Director, EMS
878 Peachtree Street, N.E.
Atlanta, GA 30309
(404) 656–6452

HAWAII

Donna Maiava
Acting Chief, EMSS Branch
Department of Health
3627 Kilauea Avenue
Room 102
Honolulu, HI 96816
(808) 735–5267

IDAHO

Paul B. Anderson
Chief, EMS Bureau
Department of Health & Welfare
450 West State Street
Boise, ID 83720
(208) 334–5994

ILLINOIS

Leslie G. Stein
Chief
Division EMS & Highway
Safety
Department of Public Health
525 West Jefferson Street

Springfield, IL 62761
(217) 785–2080

INDIANA

Donald W. Moreau
Director, EMS Commission
State Office Building
Room 315
100 North Senate Avenue
Indianapolis, IN 46204–2258
(317) 232–3980

IOWA

Donald E. Kerns
Director, EMS Section
Department of Health
Lucas State Office Building
Des Moines, IA 50319–0075
(515) 281–4962

KANSAS

Lyle E. Eckhart
Director
Bureau of EMS
111 West 6th
Topeka, KS 66603
(913) 296–7296

KENTUCKY

Ms. Pat Loar Jones
Manager, EMS
Department of Human Resources
275 East Main Street
Frankfort, KY 40601
(502) 564–8948

LOUISIANA

Albert Hecht
Administrator
Bureau of EMS
200 Lafayette Street, Suite 600
Baton Rouge, LA 70801
(504) 342–2600

MAINE

Kevin McGinnis
Director, Office of EMS
Department of Human Services
295 Water Street
Augusta, ME 04330
(207) 289–3953

MARYLAND

R. Adams Cowley, M.D.
Director, EMS-MIEMS
31 South Greene Street
Baltimore, MD 21201
(301) 328–7800

Ameen Ramzy, M.D.
Medical Director, State EMS
31 South Greene Street
Baltimore, MD 21201
(301) 328–5074

MASSACHUSETTS

Frank Keslof
Director, Office of EMS
Department of Public Health
80 Boylston Street, Suite 1040
Boston, MA 02116
(617) 451–3433

199

Alan Doelp

MICHIGAN

Thomas Lindsay
Acting Chief, Division of EMS
3500 North Logan
P.O. Box 30035
Lansing, MI 48909
(517) 335–8503

MINNESOTA

Wayne Arrowood
Acting Chief, EMS
Department of Health
717 S.E. Delaware Street
P.O. Box 9441
Minneapolis, MN 55440
(612) 623–5209

MISSISSIPPI

Wade N. Spruill, Jr.
Chief, Office of EMS
State Board of Health
P.O. Box 1700
Jackson, MS 39215–1700
(601) 960–7889

MISSOURI

Kenneth E. Cole, Jr.
Director, Bureau of EMS
State Division of Health
P.O. Box 570
Jefferson City, MO 65101
(314) 751–4022, ext. 239

MONTANA

Drew E. Dawson
Chief, EMS Bureau
Department of Health & Environmental Services
Cogswell Building
Helena, MT 59620
(406) 449–3895

NEBRASKA

Robert Leopold
Director, EMS Division
301 Centennial Mall S.
3rd Floor
Box 95007
Lincoln, NE 68509
(402) 471–2158

NEVADA

Reba L. Chappell
Chief, EMS Office
505 East King Street
Capitol Complex
Kinkead Building
Carson City, NV 89710
(702) 885–4800

NEW HAMPSHIRE

Marcia Houch
Acting Director, EMS
Health & Welfare Building
Hazen Drive
Concord, NH 03301
(603) 271–4569

NEW JERSEY

Roy W. Nickels
Director, EMS
State Department of Health
C.N. 363
Trenton, NJ 08625
(609) 292–0782

NEW MEXICO

Barak Wolff
Chief, EMS Bureau
Health & Environment Department
P.O. Box 968
Sante Fe, NM 87504–0968
(505) 827–2509

NEW YORK

Michael Gilbertson
Director
EMS Development Program
ESP Tower Building
Room 710
Albany, NY 12237
(518) 474–3171

NORTH CAROLINA

Ed Browning
Assistant Chief, Education
Office of EMS
Department of Human
Resources
701 Barbour Drive
Raleigh, NC 27603–2008
(919) 733–2285

NORTH DAKOTA

Robert P. Friese
Director, EMS Division
Department of Health
State Capitol Building
Bismarck, ND 58505
(701) 724–2388

OHIO

James Bartholomew, DDS
Director, EMS Training Office
65 South Front Street
Columbus, OH 43215
(614) 466–9447

OKLAHOMA

Gary Forbis
Director, Division of EMS
1000 N.E. 10th, Room 211
P.O. Box 53551
Oklahoma City, OK 73152
(405) 271–4062

OREGON

Nancy Clarke
Manager, EMS
State Health Department
Portland, OR 97201
(503) 229–6365

PENNSYLVANIA

S. Gail Dubs
EMS Representative

Health & Welfare Building
Room 1033
P.O. Box 90
Harrisburg, PA 17108
(717) 787-8740

RHODE ISLAND

Harold A. Pace
Chief, Division of EMS
Department of Health & Environmental Control
75 Davis Street
Providence, RI 02908

SOUTH CAROLINA

Albert M. Futrell
Director, Division of EMS
Department of Health & Environmental Control
2600 Bull Street
Columbia, SC 29201
(803) 758-8616

SOUTH DAKOTA

Robert Graff
Director, EMS Program
Department of Health
523 East Capitol
Pierre, SD 57501

TENNESSEE

Joseph B. Phillips
Director, Division of EMS
Department of Health & Environment

283 Plus Park
Nashville, TN 37219-5407
(615) 367-6259

TEXAS

Gene Weatherall
Chief
Bureau of Emergency Management
Department of Health
1100 West 49th Street
Austin, TX 78756-3199
(512) 465-2601

UTAH

Richard L. Warburton
Director, Division of EMS
Department of Health
P.O. Box 16660
Salt Lake City, UT 84116-0660
(801) 538-6435/6608

VERMONT

Dan Manz
Director, EMS
60 Main Street
Box 70
Burlington, VT 05402
(802) 863-7310

VIRGINIA

Susan D. McHenry
Director, Bureau of EMS
Department of Health
109 Governor Street

Room 1001
Richmond, VA 23219
(804) 786–5188

WASHINGTON

Howard Farley
Section Head, EMS
Division of Health
Department of Social & Health
Services
1112 South Quince Street
ET-34
Olympia, WA 98504
(206) 753–2095

WEST VIRGINIA

F. M. Cooley, M.D.
Director, Office of EMS
Department of Health
Building 3, Room 426
1800 Washington Street, East
Charleston, WV 25305
(304) 348–3956

WISCONSIN

Michael French
Chief, EMS Section
Division of Health
Box 309
Madison, WI 53701
(608) 266–0472

WYOMING

Jim Murray
Chief, EMS Program

Hathaway Building, Room 527
Cheyenne, WY 82002
(307) 777–7955

GUAM

Lydia Flores
EMS, P.O. Box 2816
Agana, GU 96910
011 (671) 734–2931, ext. 268

PUERTO RICO

Boyd Collazo, M.D.
Executive Director, EMS
G.P.O. Box 71423
San Juan, PR 00936

VIRGIN ISLANDS

Kirk Grybowski
Director, EMS
Department of Health
P.O. Box 7309
St. Thomas, VI 00801
(809) 774–9000, ext. 316

NATIONWIDE

Fran Berry
Executive Director
Natl. Assoc. of State EMS Di-
rectors
Council of State Governments
P.O. Box 11910
Lexington, KY 40578

Appendix III _____
PEDIATRIC EMS TRAINING PROGRAM GRADUATES

ALABAMA

Nancy Carlisle
254 Shenandoah Drive
Birmingham, AL 35226
(205) 934–2595

Brent Dierking
250 Old Bay Front Drive
Mobile, AL 36615
(205) 471–7298

Larry Gosdin
600 Crestview Drive
Gadsden, AL 35903
(205) 546–0484

ALASKA

Steve Iha
P.O. Box 33315
Juneau, AK 99803
(909) 789–7554

Mary Rowe
P.O. Box 806
Sitka, AK 99835
(907) 747–8005

Casie Williams
P.O. Box 671003
Chugiak, AK 99567
(907) 274–3651

ARIZONA

Barbara Aehlert
Samaritan Health Services
P.O. Box 25489
Phoenix, AZ 85002
(602) 495–4285

Patty Costa
Samaritan Health Services
P.O. Box 25489
Phoenix, AZ 85002
(602) 495–4285

Jennifer Van Kirk
Tucson Medical Center Education Center
P.O. Box 42195
Tucson, AZ 85733
(602) 327–5461

ARKANSAS

Virginia Clevenger
P.O. Box 47
Springdale, AR 72764
(501) 751–5711, ext. 281

Jo Ann Cobble
616 Alta Lane
Jacksonville, AR 72076
(501) 661–5772

Jerry Simmons
418 Tabor Street
East Camden, AR 71701
(501) 574–1521

CALIFORNIA

Carol Gallagher
3202 Marwick Avenue
Long Beach, CA 90808
(213) 533–2291

Margaret McKenna
1800 Coastline Drive, No. 10
Malibu, CA 90265
(213) 829–8218

Ron Martin
Sierra Ambulance Service
P.O. Box 49

Oakhurst, CA 93644
(209) 683–4393

Ginger Ochs
1129 Manchester
National City, CA 92050
(619) 543–6449

Luis Ponce
Tahoe City Fire Department
300 North Lake Boulevard
Tahoe City, CA 95730
(916) 583–6912

COLORADO

Janet Cunningham
4039 Newton
Denver, CO 80211
(303) 861–8888

Doug Krause
P.O. Box 2501
Vail, CO 81658
(303) 476–0855

Elizabeth Rieber
112 Sunway
Bailey, CO 80421

CONNECTICUT

William Powers
14 Ellise Road
Storrs, CT 06268
(413) 784–5167

Wendy Sawyer
Staff Development Coordinator, ER

Lawrence and Memorial Hospital
365 Montauk Avenue
New London, CT 06320
(203) 442–0711, ext. 2683

William Tinnel
6 Rhode Island Drive
Oakdale, CT 06370
(203) 526–7980

DISTRICT OF COLOMBIA

Craig DeAtley
George Washington University
School of Medicine & Health Services
2140 Pennsylvania Avenue, N.W.
Washington, DC 20037
(202) 676–4375

Danny Mott
D.C. Fire Department
1018 13th Street, N.W.
Washington, DC 20005
(202) 745–2235

DELAWARE

Bruce Truitt
R.D. 2, Box 679C
Camden, DE 19934
(302) 674–7200

FLORIDA

Nancy Jerz
6889 Sedgewick Court
Fort Myers, FL 33907

Susan Ullah
P.O. Box 1026
Fernandina Beach, FL 32034
(904) 261–7431

Richard Wiederhold
920 Gran Paso Drive
Orlando, FL 32825
(305) 299–5000

GEORGIA

Gail Lites Helmly
Rt. 1, Box 5110
Hiram, GA 30141
(404) 589–4307

David Loftin
8 Susan Wayne Center, S.W.
Rome, GA 30161
(404) 295–6187

Michael Allen McCullough
175 Johnson Avenue
Fayetteville, GA 30214
(404) 461–8111

HAWAII

Edward Kalinowski
99–427 Palaiallii Way
Aiea, HI 96701
(808) 734–9288

Helen Wexler
4970 Kilauea Avenue, #608
Honolulu, HI 96816
(808) 735–8288

Carol Ah Yo
P.O. Box 102
Honomu, HI 96728
(808) 935–8002

IDAHO

Steven Baisch
P.O. Box 2105
Twin Falls, ID 83303
(208) 737–2000

Barbara Chamberlin
1252 Cotterell Way
Boise, ID 83709
(208) 383–4427

Paul Christensen
3210 Colorado
Caldwell, ID 83605
(208) 459–4641

ILLINOIS

Michael Hansen
128 Oxford
Clarendon Hills, IL 60514
(312) 774–4550

Ronald Simpson
118 West Altgeld Avenue
Glendale Heights, IL 60139
(312) 668–4836

INDIANA

Gary Atherton
Porter Memorial Hospital
814 LaPorte Avenue

Valparaiso, IN 46383
(219) 465–4793

Noreen Broering
68508 Miami Highway
Bremen, IN 46506
(219) 237–7232

Daniel Garman
8613 Amy Lane
Indianapolis, IN 46356
(317) 232–3980

Judith Hallam
1001 West 10th Street
Indianapolis, IN 46202
(317) 630–7427

IOWA

Terri Grantham
R.R. 2, Box 229 A-5
Solon, IA 52333
(319) 398–6195

Paul Hudson
2221 Storm Street
Ames, IA 50010
(515) 239–2109

Elizabeth Wehrman
510 Walnut Court
LeClaire, IA 52753
(319) 322–1361

KANSAS

Terry Chaffee
4853 Horton

Mission, KS 66206
(913) 588–7600

Carolynn Darby Nellis
11067 Century Lane
Overland, KS 66210
(913) 469–8500, ext. 3289

Jerry Ryman
P.O. Box 206
Liberal, KS 67901
(316) 275–6109

KENTUCKY

Michael Bouvier
P.O. Box 2150
Owensboro, KY 42302
(502) 926–4520

Ralph Garvin
2216 Cedar Street
Ashland, KY 41101
(606) 325–9702

Ann Reeser
99 Timberline Court South
Elizabethtown, KY 42701

LOUISIANA

David Lawrence
4137 Laurel Street
New Orleans, LA 70115

Dwight Polk
P.O. Box 32021
Lafayette, LA 70593–2021
(318) 231–5601

MAINE

Judy Lemburg
300 Main Street
Lewiston, ME 04240
(207) 795–2874

Richard Rittenhouse
14 Central Street
Winthrop, ME 04364
(207) 289–3953

Ham Robbins
Maine EMS
295 Water Street
Augusta, ME 04330
(207) 289–3953

MARYLAND

Kenneth Brown
7931 Redjacket Way
Jessup, MD 20794
(301) 596–5135

Richard Himes
Maryland Fire & Rescue Institution
University of Maryland
College Park, MD 20740
(202) 357–2368

James Miller
Prince Georges County Fire Department
4318 Rhode Island Avenue
Brentwood, MD 20722
(301) 699–2909

Samanthia Robinson
4010 Norcross Street
Hillcrest Heights, MD 20748
(202) 745–2235

JoAnne Schultz
126 Truitt Street
Salisbury, MD 20748
(301) 548–3122

Audrey Sisson
Montgomery County Fire &
Rescue Training Academy
10025 Darnstown Road
Rockville, MD 20906
(301) 279–1834

Larry West
240 Waterstreet Road
Walkersville, MD 21793
(301) 328–3662

MASSACHUSETTS

Glenn Coffin
2 Chadwick Road
South Dennis, MA 02660
(617) 389–2242

Kenneth Leary
47 Fairfield Street
Dedham, MA 02026
(617) 653–3400

Kevin Prendergast
1 12th Avenue
Averell, MA 01830
(617) 683–4000, ext. 2517

MICHIGAN

Glenda Dolehanty
312 Fitch Street
Durand, MI 48429
(517) 288–4231

Steve Smit
2075 Brook Trails Court, S.E.
Grand Rapids, MI 49508
(616) 241–4395

MINNESOTA

Beth Adams
EMS, 701 Park Avenue South
Minneapolis, MN 55415–1676
(612) 347–5681

Mr. Lynn Boergerhoff
7374 Van Buren Street
Fridley, MN 55432
(507) 389–6419

Robert Kuchar
5122 Idlewild
Duluth, MN 55804
(218) 726–4430

MISSISSIPPI

Cheryl Adams
P.O. Box 299
Fernwood, MS 39635

Charlene Byrd
Route 2, Box 176
Seminary, MS 39479
(601) 264–4235

Gail Salyer
Rt. 1, Box 184 A
Fulton, MS 38843
(601) 862–3101, ext. 215

MISSOURI

P. Gregg Grooms
103 South 36th
St. Joseph, MO 64506

Mike Krtek
R. #3, Box 203 HH
Carthage, MO 64836
(417) 623–3348

Jimmie Tune
1341 South Pecos
Columbia, MO 65201
(314) 882–8017

MONTANA

Earl Neff
411 4th Street S.E.
Sidney, MT 59270
(406) 482–2120

Dayle Perrin
2120 Billings Avenue, #A
Helena, MT 59601
(406) 444–4895

Nels Sanddal
Critical Illness & Trauma
Foundation
P.O. Box 656
Boulder, MT 59632
(406) 225–4224

NEBRASKA

Jill Christiansen
601 South Slaughter
Pender, NE 68047

Kathy Dernovich
P.O. Box 163
Culbertson, NE 69024
(308) 345–6303

Jerrell Gerdes
1160 16th Street
Box 481
Henderson, NE 68371

NEVADA

Deena McKenzie
5455 Artemesia Road
Carson City, NV 89701
(702) 882–1361

John Mohler
180 Virgil Drive
Sparks, NV 89431
(702) 789–3154

Linda Netski
7121 Cornflower Drive
Las Vegas, NV 89128
(702) 386–9985

NEW HAMPSHIRE

Mary E. Connor
7 Westbrook Drive
Nashua, NH 03855
(603) 882–3000

Frank Hubbel
RFD #1, Box 163
Conway, NH 03818
(603) 447–6711

Wilma Low
89 Locust Street
Dover, NH 02820

NEW JERSEY

Patricia Cone
12 Preswick Drive
Medford, NJ 08055
(609) 292–6789

Nancy Kelly
P.O. Box 524
Fairfield, NJ 07022
(609) 292–6789

Kevin Monaghan
1304 Bullard Avenue
Forked River, NJ 08731
(609) 292–6789

NEW MEXICO

Ann Dunlap
P.O. Box 780
Corrales, NM 87048
(505) 277–5757

Ann Fedderson
1210 Gold, S.W.
Albuquerque, NM 87102
(505) 225–4225

Terry Landess
University of New Mexico EMS
Academy
620 Camino De Salus, N.E.
Albuquerque, NM 87131
(505) 277–5757

NEW YORK

Mark Knowles
RD #2, Box 107-B
Dexter, NY 13634
(315) 782–7400

Kevin Kraus
10 Clove Court
Clifton Park, NY 12065
(518) 474–3171

Andrew Stern
Corning Tower, Room 2270
Empire State Plaza
Albany, NY 12237
(518) 474–3171

Owen Traynor
899 A Jerusalum
Uniondale, NY 11553
(516) 785–3392

NORTH CAROLINA

Martha McCrea
Catawba Valley Community
College
Route 3, Box 283
Hickory, NC 28602–9699
(704) 327–9124

Michael Shutak
1911 Onslow Drive
Jacksonville, NC 28540
(919) 396–6760

Joyce Winstead
Rt. 3, Box 289 B
Nashville, NC 27856
(919) 399–8101

NORTH DAKOTA

Marlys Haisley
523 N.E. 2nd Street
LaMouee, ND 58458
(701) 883–5720

Thomas Ross
Med 1 300 North 7th Street
Bismarck, ND 58501
(701) 224–6075

Nadia Smetana
RR 1, Box 57
Lansford, ND 58750
(701) 857–2490

OHIO

Jamie Friery
2090 Brown
Lakewood, OH 44107
(216) 292–5381

John Mason
215 North Broadway
Medina, OH 44256
(216) 723–3231, ext. 3600

Kent Spitler
5137 Outerview Drive
Springfield, OH 45502
(513) 325–9456

Robert Wagoner
NREMT, P.O. Box 29233
Columbus, OH 43229
(614) 888–4484

OKLAHOMA

Pat Brown
Oklahoma State College
1210 North Spurgeon
Altus, OK 73521
(405) 477–2000

Russell Calhoun
8800 South Drexel, #215
Oklahoma City, OK 73159
(405) 682–7573

Robert Hawley
P.O. Box 770056
Oklahoma City, OK 73177
(405) 271–4027

OREGON

Debra Ann Lane
P.O. Box 968
Redmond, OR 97756
(503) 548–8131, ext. 280

Beverly Moore
2465 S.E. 40th Street
Albany, OR 97321
(503) 928–2361, ext. 231

Ra Wollenburg
542 Comanche Drive
Medford, OR 97501
(503) 535–4222

PENNSYLVANIA

Rod Drawbaugh
EMS Systems Coordinator
York Hospital
1001 South George Street
York, PA 17405
(717) 771–2450

George Moerkirk, M.D.
806 South 25th Street
Allentown, PA 18103
(215) 776–8600

Terry Scott
Box 9
Chalk Hill, PA 15419

Karen Smith
35 Winchester Gardens
Carlisle, PA 17013
(717) 782–3590

RHODE ISLAND

Gary Kleinman
1776 Bicentennial Way, #0–7
North Providence, RI 02911
(401) 863–3671

Mark Levesque
53 Andrews Street
Woonsocket, RI 02895
(401) 769–4142

Karen Mignone
419 Nayatt Road
Barrington, RI 02806
(914) 993–0918

SOUTH CAROLINA

Frances Hansen
6915 Nursery Road
Columbia, SC 29210
(803) 765–6392

Janice G. Johnson
7013 John Edward Street
Columbia, SC 29209
(803) 794–3940

William Mastrianni
121 Hunt Club Drive
Summerville, SC 29483
(803) 763–9224

SOUTH DAKOTA

Stan Hope
Indian Health Services
3823 Clifton
Rapid City, SD 57702
(605) 348–1900, ext. 267

Mark McCabe
114 East Nevada
Rapid City, SD 57701
(605) 341–3100

Nancy Ramesbothom
524 South Glendale
Sioux Falls, SD 57104
(605) 333–1000

David Snavely
523 East Capitol
Pierre, SD 57501
(605) 773-3737

TENNESSEE

David Ashburn
EMS Center of Excellence
Volunteer State Community
College
Nashville Pike
Gallatin, TN 37066-3188
(615) 452-8600
(800) 323-4220

Richard Collier
1908 Convent Pl. #4
Nashville, TN 37212
(615) 452-8605, ext. 236
(615) 741-3215, ext. 202

Brent Lemonds
412 Lambuth Boulevard
Jackson, TN 38301
(901) 424-3520

TEXAS

Martha Libby
1407 Deer Trace Drive
Cedar Park, TX 78613
(512) 469-2050

Stephen Marshall
8007 Claret
Amarillo, TX 79110
(806) 358-7111, ext. 31

Paul Tabor
9815 Copper Creek Drive
#1123
Austin, TX 78729
(512) 465-2601

UTAH

DeAnn Barnson
8690 Scottish Drive
Sandy, UT 84092
(801) 943-1518

Evelyn Draper
2360 East 6200 South
Ogden, UT 84403
(801) 626-6521

Laurie Storey
426 North Orchard Drive, #12
No. Salt Lake City, UT 84054
(801) 521-1316

VIRGINIA

James Alderton
Fairfax County Fire & Rescue
Department
4031 University Drive
Fairfax, VA 22030
(703) 631-8121

Donna Burns
University of Virginia Medical
Center
Charlottesville, VA 22908
(804) 924-8484

Judith Cauley
P.O. Box 58
Troutville, VA 24175
(703) 981–7556

Steven Strawderman
12540 Basswood Drive
Manassas, VA 22111
(703) 335–6800

VERMONT

Joe Golden
60 Main Street, Box 70
Burlington, VT 05402
(802) 863–7310

Steve Hazleton
EMT Training Director
Rutland Regional Medical Center
Rutland, VT 05701
(802) 775–7111, ext. 450

Mike O'Keefe
134 Pearl Street
Essex Junction, VT 05452

WASHINGTON

Paul Berlin
11105 37th Avenue, N.W.
Gig Harbor, WA 98335
(206) 756–5164

Murray Gordon
8906 10th Drive, S.E.
Everett, WA 98208
(206) 259–8709

Richard Kness
East 12123 25th Street
Spokane, WA 99206
(509) 456–2694

WEST VIRGINIA

Leah Heimbach
215 East Main Street, #A
Bridgeport, WV 26330
(304) 366–8764

Paul Seamann
900 Ewart Avenue
Beckley, WV 25801
(304) 253–8469

Louis Vargo
R.D. #2
Rayland, OH 43943
(304) 243–3344

WISCONSIN

Ramona Atkinson, R.N.
N7282 Caberg Coulee Road
Holmen, WI 54636
(608) 785–0530, ext. 3267

Michael Milbrath
4046 North 84th Street
Milwaukee, WI 53222
(414) 257–6736

June Winnie
409 Radtke Street
Schofield, WI 54476
(715) 847–2121

WYOMING

Douglas Follick
1024 North Elma
Casper, WY 82601
(307) 577-2102/2426

Margaret Leininger
1400 Uinta Drive
Green River, WY 82935
(307) 875-6010

Scott Paris
311 Bluebell Lane
P.O. Box A
Worland, WY 82401
(307) 347-4592

GUAM

Christine Gyulavics
P.O. Box 21543 GMF

Barrigada, GU 96921
(671) 646-8801 or
(671) 472-8911, ext. 318

David Peredo
P.O. Box 22835 GMF
Marianas Island, GU 96921
(671) 472-8911, ext. 343

VIRGIN ISLANDS

David Sweeney
P.O. Box 520
Christiansted
St. Croix, VI 00840
(809) 773-1311

Alexander Williams
P.O. Box 3611
4-1-23 Estate Fortuna
Charlotte Amalie, VI
(809) 776-8311, ext. 176

Appendix IV _____

PEDIATRIC HOSPITALS:

CANADA

Alberta Children's Provincial
General Hospital
1820 Richmond Road
South West
Calgary, Alberta
T2T 5C7
(403) 229–7211

Children's Hospital
4480 Oak Street
Vancouver, British Columbia
V6H 3V4
(604) 875–2345

Health Sciences Centre
800 Sherbrook Street
Winnipeg, Manitoba
R3A 1M4
(204) 774–6511

Izaak Walton Killam Hospital
for Children
5850 University Avenue
Halifax, Nova Scotia
B3J 3G9
(902) 428–8111

Children's Hospital of
Eastern Ontario
401 Smyth Road
Ottawa, Ontario
K1H 8L1
(613) 737–7600

The Hospital for Sick Children
555 University Avenue
Toronto, Ontario
M5G 1X8
(416) 597–1500

Children's Hospital of
Western Ontario
800 Commissioners Road East
London, Ontario
N6A 4G5
(519) 681–6711

L'Hôspital de Montŕeal
pour Enfants
2300 rue Tupper
Montreal, Quebec
H3H 1P3
(514) 934–4400

Alan Doelp

University Hospital
Saskatoon, Saskatchewan
S7N 0X0
(306) 244–2323

Walter McKenzie Centre
8440 112 Street
Edmonton, Alberta
T6G 2B7
(403) 432–8822

About the Author_____

ALAN DOELP has a background in both print and broadcast journalism; a former *Baltimore Sun* reporter, he is presently vice-president and managing editor of PressNet Systems, Inc., an electronic news service. He also dabbles in politics, computers, cabinetmaking, and air-compressor repair. This is his fourth book of medical nonfiction.